Take Charge
of Your
HEALTH

Take Charge of Your HEALTH

of Your

The Guide to Personal Health Competence

PETER WAYS, M.D.

The Stephen Greene Press
Lexington, Massachusetts

First published in 1985 by The Stephen Greene Press, Inc.
Published simultaneously in Canada by Penguin Books Canada Limited
Distributed by Viking Penguin Inc., 40 West 23rd Street, New York, New York 10010

LIBRARY OF CONGRESS CATALOGING IN PUBLICATION DATA
Ways, Peter, 1928–
   Take charge of your health.
   Bibliography: p.
   Includes index.
   1. Health.   2. Nutrition.   3. Exercise.
4. Holistic medicine.   5. Physician and patient.   I. Title.
RA776.W35   1985   613   84-21151
ISBN 0-8289-0548-7

Printed in the United States of America by
Hamilton Printing Company, Rensselaer, N.Y.
Designed by Irving Perkins Associates

The illustrations on pages 114 and 226–229 are by Jacqueline Ropski-Konkol of Chicago.

*This book is dedicated with love and appreciation
to my parents, Dorothea and Max, who nurtured my
creativity, valued my curiosity, and let me take risks.*

Acknowledgments

THERE are many people without whose help, goading and inspiration this book would have never been written. I am grateful to them all. Long before I set pen to paper my daughters Heather and Carol Ways awakened me to alternative modes of healing, an awareness which augmented a burgeoning interest in health rather than sickness. My soulmate, Karen Johnson, encouraged me to write rather than only talk about a book, and she has given me continuing support and valuable criticism. Larry Hulbert, friend and colleague, read an ancient draft in its entirety, then helped me face its gross inadequacies and begin again. He also reviewed parts of later versions and offered his incisive comments with quantities of vital encouragement. Another daughter, Martha Ways, made important comments on numerous chapters and (aided and abetted by Karen) broadened my perspective on key aspects of women's health.

While I was writing this book my son Peter often stimulated me by asking tough questions, and by his shining and vigorous passage from adolescence to adulthood. Watching my friends Jan and Ed Romond following the sudden and tragic death of their young son Mark helped me learn more about emotional-spiritual growth and strength.

Max Ways, my father, is a writer. Five years ago he suffered a stroke. Despite significant difficulties with his speech and the act of writing, he has time and again read and incisively critiqued the concepts and tone of the manuscript. In so doing his intellectual integrity has enriched my own. Clem Brown, Rosemary McConkey and Barry Rosen have inspired me by visibly practicing health maintenance and holistic medicine with their clients. Barry, Sally Rubenstone, Peter Finkelstein and Barrie Cowan have given many helpful suggestions about the manuscript as well as their love and encouragement. A position paper by Sally on nutrition awakened me to the serious issues involved in the depletion and alteration of food. Dale Alexander was of enormous help outlining and providing content for Chapter 11. It could not have been done without him. Matthew Kiel provided substantial assistance in rewriting Chapter 4. I am grateful to the following friends and colleagues who read and critiqued one or more chapters: John Engel, Connie Filling, Marcia Lipetz, Cynthia and Joe DeFors, Jan Romond, Marta Erin and Barbara Sharf.

Last but far from least the debt to Tom Begner, my editor, is great. He believed that Personal Health Competence was an important and interesting concept. Later he did expert and necessary surgery on the manuscript. The managing editor, Kathy Shulga, and the copy editor, Margaret McCauley, made many helpful suggestions on the text. Kathy and her staff have shepherded the manuscript through design and production to become a real book.

Contents

Acknowledgments   vii

Part I: THE WHAT AND WHY OF PERSONAL HEALTH COMPETENCE   1

1. About Personal Health Competence   7

Part II: THE PATHWAY OF HEALTH ACCOUNTING AND INFORMATION GATHERING   15

2. Taking Your Inventory of Health, Well-Being, and Problems   17

3. Your Personal Health Guide   33

4. The Self-Health Record: Keeping Track   41

5. Gathering and Describing Health Information   52

Part III: THE PATHWAY OF EMOTIONAL-SPIRITUAL HEALTH   61

6. The Mind-Body Connection   63

7. Individual Emotional-Spiritual Health   72

8. Healthy Relationships   83

9. Advocacy and People-Support Systems   95

Part IV: THE PATHWAY
OF EATING, MOVING,
AND HABITS   103

10. Changing Unhealthy
Habits   105

11. Healthy Body Structure
Through Alignment,
Flexibility, and Muscle
Balance   113

12. Body Movement
and Conditioning   123

13. Eating Poorly,
Eating Well   134

14. Body Fat and
Weight Management   144

Part V: THE PATHWAY OF
ILLNESS AND
PROBLEM CARE   155

15. The Person-Doctor
Relationship: Present
Reality, Future Hope 157

16. The Person-Doctor
Relationship and How
It Works (or Doesn't) 163

17. The Beliefs and
Skills of Health
Partnership   172

18. Finding and Getting
Started with a New
Physician (or Starting
Over with Your
Old One)   184

19. The Office Visit,
Being Your Own
Specialist, Phoning the
Doctor   191

20. Alternatives to
Conventional Therapy:
Why Not?   198

21. Being in the
Hospital   207

22. Your Journey, Your
Health   214

Appendix A. The Lifetime
Health-Monitoring Plan
of Breslow and Somers   218

Appendix B. Status of
Various States on Patient
Access to Medical Records 224

Appendix C. One Dependable
Flexibility and Muscle
Balance Routine   226

General Resources   232

Index   235

Take Charge
of Your
HEALTH

Part I

THE WHAT AND WHY OF PERSONAL HEALTH COMPETENCE

OUR society provides everyone the opportunity of becoming good at certain things, whether in work or play — things like writing, reading, basic mathematics, driving a car, or typing. However, we are not given much opportunity to acquire skills in maintaining and valuing our health. We are neither encouraged nor required to accept responsibility for our health nor to learn the skills and perspectives for staying healthy, enriching that healthiness and dealing more effectively with medical problems when they occur. We do acknowledge the fundamental and immeasurable value of enduring health. Almost everyone will say that his or her most valuable assets are a healthy body and mind, but neither parents, churches, workplace, nor schools make a commitment to provide the necessary "health competence" in a *systematic* way. That is not to say that people do not learn things about how to take care of themselves. They certainly do. Regular tooth brushing and the recent boom in running are important examples. But basic *Personal Health Competence* is not systematically learned.

Not too long ago a book called *Personal Health Competence* would have focused on how to care for yourself when sick, how to endure the hospital experience without undue suffering, what should be in your home medicine cabinet, and some first aid. And a few years ago not many people would have thought twice about that book's limitations. Today, however, such a book could not be called *Personal Health Competence*. The reason is simple: in the last decade our concept of health has been greatly enriched.

An anecdote from my own past reveals how much our concepts of health have broadened. My second year in medical school was demanding and anxiety-provoking. Halfway through the year, I began to have tightness and pressure in

1

my throat and difficulty swallowing. I was uncomfortable and scared. The physician in the health service listened to my story and examined my throat. "Don't see much — tonsils aren't very large. Let's just watch it for a week." My tonsils had been removed when I was six, but the doctor said, "Sometimes they grow back." The week passed without change, so I was sent to an ear, nose, and throat professor who looked at my throat, and said, "Those tonsils need to come out." "But," I said, "they were removed once." "Well," he replied, "they need to come out again." As both medical student and patient, I was intimidated by this august professor. No more was said. The surgery was scheduled.

The fourth-year student assigned to the ear, nose, and throat services was a friend. After his interview and examination he thought I was suffering from globus hystericus, a condition caused by tension and anxiety and completely unrelated to tonsils or any other "organic" medical problem. The resident physician on the service agreed. Neither the student nor the resident told me about the diagnosis (which I now know as obvious and correct) until *after* the surgery. Neither suggested that the unnecessary operation be cancelled! Neither spoke to the professor.

The first lesson of this story relates to personal responsibility for health and medical well-being. I was a reasonably adult and assertive individual who was *part* of the system and possessed far more knowledge than the average consumer. However, I was *not meaningfully involved* in the decision to operate. Painful major surgery with potentially serious complications was the result. I was not at all convinced that surgery was the best therapy or even necessary. My tonsils had already been removed (incompletely removed in the first place, they had indeed "grown back," although they were still small as tonsils go). Neither the difficulty swallowing nor the pressure felt close to the tonsils. One did not seem like a likely explanation of the other. Yet I had been steeped for years in the attitude that you don't question the doctor. I was unable to ask the right questions or raise pertinent objections. This was an authoritarian physician-patient transaction. Commonplace in 1951, this domination by the doctor is changing only slowly. Even today my story is repeated thousands of times a day in physicians' offices and hospitals. You can probably think of an experience that embodied some of the same physician-patient dynamics for you.

The second lesson of the story is that the physicians involved were uncomfortable in the face of emotional illness. Perhaps, you think, they made an honest error; I believe not. I attended a good medical school. Globus hystericus is frightening and uncomfortable for the patient, but easy to diagnose. With reassurance and some ventilation of the underlying anxieties, the symptom usually subsides in a few weeks. I'm sure that both the health service physician and the ENT professor knew about globus hystericus and how to treat it. Admittedly, 30-year hindsight may be foolhardy, but I view both the decision to refer me and the one to operate on a pair of insignificant tonsillar tabs as evidence of their discomfort and lack of skill in acknowledging and managing emotionally induced illness.

Equally profound was my own reluctance to face the question of emotional upset or illness. Several years before, in college, after taking a battery of psycho-logical tests as part of an experiment, I was advised to have psychotherapy. I adamantly refused, although I knew from my own reactions during the psycho-logical tests that the suggestion was a sound one. Before my tonsil operation, the health service physician had explored, clumsily, but definitely, the possibility that the stress and tension of medical school might be a contributing factor to my symptoms. I also knew then that there was substance in his concern. I again re-fused to *own* the possibility of emotional upset and wouldn't be involved in that discussion. Even after surgery when I accepted the fact that I had suffered from globus hystericus, I was unwilling to enter a counseling or therapeutic relation ship which might have benefited me. Thus, the defenses against acknowledging emotional illness were not only operating for the doctors, but also for me, the patient.

The choice of surgery as the therapeutic modality speaks directly to a third les-son. Surgery was inappropriate, in fact, not indicated. Surgery of any kind under general anesthesia involves significant risk or complications and occasionally death. Globus hystericus itself has no potential for death or disability. You might say that surgery under these conditions was negligent malpractice. More likely it was cultural practice. For several decades medical practitioners have indulged a propensity to find a pill or surgical solution for every problem rather than enter-tain other alternatives. Since none of our present-day tranquilizers were avail-able, surgery was selected.

So, a lack of self-responsibility for one's own health and medical affairs, disin-clination of physicians and patients to deal with emotional illness, and the propensity to find a pill or surgical solution for every problem are all issues brought into focus by my "tonsil" story.

Still another characteristic of our medical/health care system which also has important bearing on the concept of health and health competence is not illus-trated by the story. Like the others, it is deeply rooted in the process of my own medical education and training, and that of all physicians in practice today. Our training and orientation was exclusively in manifest disease—abnormal situations in which organ or organ system derangement was clearly evident. Such condi-tions were intriguing to diagnose, challenging to treat, and provided unusual re-search opportunities for faculty. Certainly this preoccupation has hastened progress against disease. But as a result, physicians practicing today have had es-sentially no encouragement or training in *health maintenance, disease preven-tion,* and the *fostering of well-being* (wellness). Not only have they not been encouraged and trained to do this for their patients, too few value their own health maintenance and emotional and physical well-being!

Certainly, until about 12 years ago, I paid little attention to my own health. Oh, I did not like being sick (although sometimes it clearly had its benefits); I just didn't think much about health as a personal resource that could be nur-tured, maintained, and even expanded. Consequently, I didn't think about the personal frame of mind and the skills which might help people do that for themselves. Then, within four years I suffered two herniated (slipped) disks in my lower spine, both of which resulted in back surgery, and developed high blood pressure (hypertension) which required treatment with drugs. Then it all came together for me. I realized that I could have avoided both the back problems and the hypertension had I practiced different habits and ways of living. Furthermore, it was clear that millions of medical problems in this country could be avoided or minimized by applying analogous good health maintenance practices. Such habits and life-style components are now part of what I call *health competence*. Few people in this country care well for themselves. In fact, we are often subtly but systematically encouraged *not* to do so. Witness the messages to which young people are regularly exposed. It is okay to smoke, drink alcohol, be significantly overweight, be inactive, drive unsafely, and eat salty, sugary, high-fat foods. Such messages are seldom spoken in so many words, but they are acted out and implied, day by day, week by week, year by year. They are powerful. Both young people and adults are consistently exposed to products, advertising, TV drama, and newspapers which depict smoking and drinking as "gusty" and sometimes glamorous. Fast, unsafe driving is part of every TV crime drama, and when have you seen someone on a TV serial putting their seat belt on? The repetitive daily diet of crime, infidelity, dishonesty, and violence on our emotional and spiritual health must be devastating. Not only are salty, sugary, high-fat foods "alright" to eat, they are constantly available. Healthy foods are advertised primarily to the groups who are already using them. In large supermarkets, the counter displaying fresh vegetables may be no longer than the candy and cookie counters combined.

Most Americans have still not accepted the fact that *their own choices about life-style and habits and the beliefs underlying them are the major factors affecting their health.* I believe this lack of acceptance is partly because they invest the physician with so much power. Consumers exercise very little self-determination when under a doctor's care—just as I did not in the tonsil story. Many decisions are made when you see your doctor for the diagnosis and management of an illness: How extensive should the interview and physical exam be? How much lab work should be ordered? Should the condition be treated with medicine or in some other way? Is surgery or some other invasive procedure indicated? Most of these decisions influence your well-being and pocketbook. But you seldom take part in them. This is an intriguing, curious, and largely unhelpful feature of our medical care system.

It is all the more important and intriguing because it is now abundantly clear that what *we* do, our personal habits and life-style vis-a-vis eating, exercise, smoking, seat belts, and health checks, has much more impact on our long-term health than what our physician does to, for, or against us. *Your health is in your hands.*

Our changing concepts of health and well-being have given rise to a number of descriptive terms: health maintenance, health promotion, wellness, well-being, and health competence, my own term. They are all important and related.

"Health promotion" and "health maintenance" mean the same thing.[1] They involve practices which keep people from getting sick. They include classical preventive medicine tools like immunization as well as changes in habits and life-style which both reduce the risk of getting certain diseases and enhance well-being. "Wellness" (or wellness medicine) and "well-being" may also be used interchangeably. They are the next level beyond health maintenance, i.e., a state of enriched or positive health. Here the individual not only takes steps to avoid sickness but works to become more complete, to extend the limits of her or his emotional, spiritual, physical, and intellectual capabilities, to integrate them with one another, and to extend caring energy to other people.

"Personal Health Competence" (PHC) is the *approaches* (or methods) *and skills* which you need to maintain optimum health (like how to eat wisely), increase your well-being (like self-awareness) and participate effectively in your own care when you are ill or injured (like using an advocate). The successful acquisition and advancement of these skills requires certain underlying beliefs (like, "I am the most important person with respect to my health"). These beliefs are, therefore, also a part of PHC. I have, for conceptual reasons and effectiveness, separated the work of becoming health competent into four *pathways*. Each of them is discussed in subsequent parts of the book.

In addition to the terms just defined, another used frequently is "holistic" or "holistic health." This term most often means complete health, health which pays attention to the mind and the spirit as well as to the body. Holistic health is the result of becoming health competent. Holistic health is the desired state; health competence is the beliefs and skills that will get you there.

Finally, in terms of definitions, it is important to signify that, for me, emotional and spiritual health are closely intertwined, if not the same. Whole health builds and grows in proportion to our awareness and healthy processing of feelings and to the extent we allow our spiritual energy to become part of everyday awareness and functioning. People who are truly well have serenity, deep faith, and an abiding connection with or belief in some Energy or Higher Power, which only some call God. Consequently, in this book, I use the term emotional-spiritual health, and I talk about a person's affect-spirit.

As others have pointed out, health maintenance and well-being, also called simply health and wellness, involve attention to present and future environmental hazards and social and community issues as well as to personal issues. This book will deal only with the latter, but not because the others are unimportant. For some people they may even be more important than the personal issues. For a coal miner, the single most important determinant of health may be the precautions the mining company takes to ventilate and purify the air which he breathes below ground. Most simply, in health it is sensible to start at home. By taking care of ourselves, coming to peace with ourselves, dealing with our own joys, conflicts, shortcomings and strengths, we become best equipped to set about

---

1. Some would argue that health promotion is a more inclusive term which encompasses some wellness activities as well as health maintenance.

working on the other things. So, given the limitations of space and time, the environmental and social issues which impinge on health will not be discussed here.

So this book is about basic Personal Health Competence. It explains what it is, what it will do for you, and how you can attain it. It will help everyone assess their own degree of health competence and increase it. You are already health competent in some ways. I know this because I have learned by watching people and teaching them that practically everyone does some positive things for their health. Some of those accomplishments are remarkable, some commonplace, but everyone seems to do something. You may already be exercising or restricting your intake of fats and highly salted foods or in psychotherapy. Every person must begin where he or she is but can progress as far as he or she wishes. It is your choice: whatever your current status, it is possible to improve upon it because only a few people are health competent to the remarkable extent possible for most of us.

Finally, inescapably, this is also a book about me. It embodies my experience as a teacher, scientist, physician, lover, spouse, athlete, writer, patient, father, and particularly the experience *of myself* as a changing and evolving person. I believe we are all here to grow — for the rest of our lives. Some say the lessons and the "exams" become harder as we get older. I'm not sure about that, and it really doesn't matter. What's clear is that most of us stop growing. This book is to help you keep on growing. As a friend recently said, "We don't need to burn out or burn up; we just need to keep burning on."

1

About Personal Health Competence

PERSONAL Health Competence (PHC). Personal — it is yours and it is unique. Your way of moving along the pathways of health competence has been and will be different from anyone else's. Health, not Medical — the goal is positive health, not simply the ability to care for yourself when ill, though that is an important part of it. Competence — the ability to perform effectively and with skill.

This chapter briefly outlines the "curriculum" or "course of study" whereby one attains health competence. Inferences about how the health competent person looks or behaves is possible and many examples are given, but *the* health competent individual will not be described because that is different for everybody.

HEALTH BELIEFS AND HEALTH COMPETENCE

Your health is closely related to your long-term habits and behaviors. Underlying those behaviors are your beliefs about health and medical care, e.g., "If I'm sick it's up to doc to fix me," or "It's just a matter of bad luck (fate) when I get sick." Health beliefs are an essential factor in the initiation and persistence of habits like smoking. They also affect how you behave with your physician and how you *feel* about and define health and illness. Most important, they determine the extent to which you *participate* in your own healing and prevent or minimize disease and medical problems in your future.

The essential foundation for a program of personal health competence is a congruent system of health beliefs. From them a person's PHC derives its vitality and maintains momentum.

People are programmed with respect to health beliefs. Certain stimulae give predictable responses. Often we are not aware of the extent to which our beliefs determine our everyday behavior. Most programs make it difficult to clearly see alternatives. People who are "on" their programs are not making choices; they are responding automatically. That's the bad news. The good news is that we can change our programs. The biggest part of that task is to acknowledge how powerfully they influence our behavior. Once this is done, we realize that *we have choices.*

Health beliefs are not only powerful, they are acquired early in life. Not long ago, I helped 22 first graders learn about their bodies and their health, and encouraged them to discuss their experiences and feelings about doctors, dentists, and hospitals. As a dividend, I ferreted out some of their beliefs about medicine and health.

The first day I asked, "Who do you think is the most important person as far as your health is concerned?" A lot of hands shot up. I called on Magen first. "The doctor," she said. Jonathan, a Chicano boy with a sad/glad face, gave the same reply. The first five people I called on all gave the same answer — "the doctor."

I reacted positively but not affirmatively. "Can anyone think of someone besides the doctor who might be the most important person in keeping you well? Mark, who do you think?" "Well, maybe the nurse." Bonnie, a saucy Oriental lady, agreed. Then came the suggestion, from Aaron, that it might be the policeman, and we discussed that. Liz then said she thought it must be the firemen because they save our homes from fire. The dentist got votes too!

While pleased with these answers and fascinated by the attitudes they conveyed, I had still not heard the one *I* thought was the most important. In answer to my dilemma, the smallest person in the class raised her hand. "Hi, what's your name?" I asked. "Eisha," she replied in a very small voice. "Well, Eisha, what do you say?" "Well," she said, "we are."

"Stop! Did everyone hear that?" I said. At last had come the response that I had hoped for. "No matter what the doctor or the nurse, or the policeman or the fireman does, it will make little difference unless you do the work." The class listened attentively. Before we ended the session that day, I asked them to respond together to the question. "Who's the most important person as far as your health is concerned?" "WE ARE," came the unanimous reply. Maybe some tapes had begun to change!

Many of our programs originate early in life and rerun so often that erasing them is difficult. Sometimes it is impossible. But younger people are more willing to change their programs and more open to new ideas. The first graders were receptive to alternative answers. My status as a physician and teacher and my willingness to reward an answer other than "the doctor" gave me a lot of power. For many of those children, this was sufficient to change their belief.

Here are six health beliefs of Personal Health Competence. All of them are fundamental.

1. You have primary responsibility for your health.
2. We human beings are holistic; body, intellect, and affect-spirit strive to function as a single unit.
3. Health is more than just the absence of disease, injury, or other problems.
4. There are valuable alternatives to contemporary western medicine with its pills, surgery, and sophisticated technology.

5. Learning and change vis-a-vis health is a process of disciplined attention to the tasks at hand, not a series of isolated instructional episodes.
6. When they occur, we can learn and grow as a result of illness, emotional problems, or other adversities.

You have primary responsibility for your health

To a highly significant degree, it is possible for you to practice self-determination and to be involved in virtually all aspects of your health and medical care. This is desirable and essential if you are to grow in health competence.

Consider the following question: "If you get sick, do you believe it is *primarily a matter of fate* (destiny, God's will) or that *you have a great deal to do with it?*" Many people reflect the attitude that their illnesses are primarily a matter of fate, but adherence to this belief means you do not accept responsibility for your health or sickness: that you concur with the idea you have little to do with whether you get ill or not in the first place, and that you have little involvement in the decisions made in the course of diagnosing and treating sickness or injury. Your will to recover from illness may be weakened.

In contrast, the belief that you *are* responsible for your health has great power. Operating from this belief is more likely to lead you to healthy habits, avoiding unhealthy ones, and increasing your well-being. Further, you will be empowered with appreciable influence on the course and severity of illness when it does occur. This happens in two ways: first, by being actively involved in the decisions which must be made in diagnosis and treatment; second, by acknowledging what you can do to care for yourself — both in terms of concrete activities (like changing diet or doing excercises to strengthen an injured leg) and as the

channel for that intangible spiritual energy which hastens and enriches the healing process.

This *acceptance* of your responsibility and impact is called *owning* your health. Such ownership is a basic "requirement" for attaining health competence. It does *not* mean that other factors are not at work, that you are always entirely responsible for whatever the problem is. It does *not* mean that you can't get support in resolving your illness or increasing your well-being. It *does* mean that your body-mind played a significant role in the genesis of the illness, the unhealthy habituation, or the failure to exercise, *and* that you must make the change if change is to be made.

People who do not accept responsibility for their health and medical care often put themselves psychologically in the hands of the physician. "Physicians are all powerful." "The doctor should have sole responsibility for medical decisions." "I'll do whatever doc suggests." These attitudes have major implications.

One implication is that people give up significant participation and decision making in their own health and healing. Their welfare *is* in the hands of their physician. They are vulnerable to poor care and automatic decision making. They also become vulnerable to any doctor who is not healthy himself, who smokes, drinks, doesn't exercise, or is overweight. More likely than not, this physician gives neither time nor investment in his practice to health maintenance and prevention. He may give very good advice while obviously not living the same game. This is not very persuasive.

In contrast, you may believe (and if you don't today then I hope this book will persuade you) that your physician is merely an expert whose job is to help you make decisions. If so, you are asserting your own primacy, control and power vis-a-vis your medical and health affairs. You are in a position of effectiveness and strength! You have accepted your responsibility.

The fact that self-responsibility is a cornerstone of health competence should not be used to "blame the victim." To accept responsibility for self requires relative freedom to choose. For example, a 17-year old woman with two parents and close friends who smoke cannot always perceive the choice not to smoke. The black ghetto youngster whose environment is steeped in poverty and crime may not perceive *not* stealing as a good choice.

Part of the process of helping people move to well-being is helping them become freer to make choices — to own their choices. This may be very difficult. People must not be blamed for their own situation if they have never had the opportunity to see a way out.

We human beings are wholistic; body, intellect, and affect-spirit strive to function as a single unit

This belief is fundamental to health competence. A healthy view of the person demands not only that we stop talking about a diseased liver or a pain in the belly (and instead talk about the person in whom the trouble occurs) but also that we never forget the profound connections between intellect, body, and affect-spirit. One of the reasons that good food, exercise, meditation, and yoga are all health-giving activities that increase our well-being is that they impact both our bodies and our minds.

This body-mind connection, as I call it, prefers unified function. Thus, there is no such thing as a purely physical act or disease, and there are few, if any, emotions or spiritual activities, stresses, or crises which do not have their reflections in our bodies.

Health is more than just the absence of disease, injury, or other problems

What is that "more?" It goes by many names: health promotion, health maintenance, prevention, wellness medicine, wellness and well-being (see Introduction for discussion of terminology). For me it makes most sense to talk about *health maintenance* and *well-being*. Together they are the "what's more."

Health maintenance involves standard immunizations and the appropriate kinds of periodic health checks by your doctor. It also includes things done by the community which we all take for granted (pure water, sewage disposal, licensing of restaurants, to name some). Beyond these things, however, it includes the behaviors we adopt to prevent disease which we know we are susceptible to. Fastening your seat belt is also an act of health maintenance, as is restricting fat in your diet to help prevent heart disease and probably breast cancer. Health maintenance is whatever you do that will help decrease the likelihood that you will develop an illness or problem in the future.

Well-being or wellness has several key aspects. The first is a *willingness to change and grow* — an antipathy to sameness, to being stuck (at least for very long). Another aspect is *wholeness*. The various aspects of your life are interconnected, not lived in isolated compartments (family, home, work, marriage, fitness). Running or walking to work is a way of connecting physical conditioning to your work; having your teenager periodically spend a day with you at your job is a way of *connecting* work and family. A third aspect is *discipline*, the pursuit of a goal (like eating wisely) with commitment and regularity. You give certain goals or activities high priority and work to attain them. Then, there is *harmony* with one's fellow people and environment. Wherever they are, healthy people find a way of being citizens not strangers. They complement situations rather than complicate them.

Finally, there is an almost magical quality to wellness or well-being for which adequate description is elusive. It involves a kind of rhythm and flow to life. Periods of intensity and dedication are followed by periods of relaxation and contemplation. Usually these cycles are major in length with minor ones superimposed. The daily cycle has these characteristics, but when a number of weeks are viewed together the rhythms will characterize the longer time span as well. This may be why running has become so popular. It has restored our rhythm. Because it is rhythmic and energetic activity, it generates a tempo which contrasts with the tempo of the rest of the day, both mentally and physically.

There are alternatives to contemporary western medicine with its pills, surgery, and other sophisticated technology

The education and practice of our physicians is basically focused on abnormalities of structure and function, and medicines and surgery are the pillars of therapy. Most office visits to the physician result in a prescription. Surgery is widely employed for many problems. Many of medicine's accomplishments have been remarkable. However, the expanded notion of health, i.e., health maintenance, increased well-being, and even the successful management of many medical care problems are often better served by certain alternative modalities (relaxation techniques, massage, meditation, good nutrition).

The dramatic technical advances of medicine are overplayed. Whenever there is a reasonable chance (and too often when there is only a slight chance) that a new breakthrough will cure something, it is given premature and inappropriate publicity. In a few instances (penicillin, the Salk vaccine), the eventual outcomes have justified their publicity, but in many more they have been relatively disappointing.

Coronary by-pass is now almost the commonest adult operation in males. Almost 200,000 are performed each year. The procedure is a remarkable technical feat and has some positive benefits. However, most of the patients involved have encouraged and accelerated their own disease by indulging certain habits which increased their risks for the underlying process of coronary arteriosclerosis. If they had adhered to an alternative diet and exercised regularly instead of being sedentary, they probably would not have required surgery.

The alternative to coronary by-pass surgery in those who now "need" it has not yet been adequately tried. We do not know whether those same people on a disciplined regimen of exercise, diet, and stress reduction might not have done equally well.

And there are many other conditions for which pills or surgery are recommended almost routinely and for which alternative therapies exist. They have not all been evaluated as well as they need to be, but health competence requires, at the least, an openness to their potential usefulness and a willingness to try them under the appropriate circumstances.

Learning and change vis-a-vis health is a process of disciplined attention to the task(s) at hand, not a series of isolated instructional episodes

The "process" involves a repetitive cycle of personal assessment, stating values and goals, the clarification of alternatives, making choices, carrying through on them, and monitoring and evaluating progress and outcomes.

The emphasis is not on what you *know*, but on what you *do* with what you know and *how* you do it. This includes the ability to see when you need further information and how to acquire it. It means that the approach or way you go about doing things is more important than the exact amount of information you have and can recall when asked.

We can learn and grow as a result of illness, emotional problems, or other adversities

Sickness is not solely a negative force. Many believe you should get well in any way you can and get on with your business. However, you may be paying little or no heed to the life circumstances out of which the illness came. You may be uninvolved in the medical decision-making and thereby accept prescriptive therapies rather than ones which might be more appropriate to your particular circumstances.

Obviously no one likes being ill. But, as the Sioux Indians say, "Illness is a teacher." In the framework of that adage each illness, injury, or problem embodies a message. They try to tell us something about how our lifestyle or environment (human, air, water, living, community) is affecting us.

A wonderful example of recognizing and heeding this lesson occurred recently. A good friend consulted me about recurrent bouts of abdominal cramps, sometimes accompanied by loose stools. After eliciting a few more details I asked him what he thought was going on. Unlike a lot of people who would have said, "Flu maybe," or "You tell me; that's what I'm here for," he was thoughtful and then answered, "Well, ever since I stopped smoking four months ago, I've been stuffing my body pretty indiscriminately with food, a lot of meat, almost anything that comes along... I suspect that has a lot to do with it." We discussed further details and then together decided on modifications in his diet (less meat, more fiber, more vegetables, less fat) which might be less provocative to his bowel. After following this regimen for a few weeks he was without symptoms.

When you regard illness as a teacher,

it becomes a means of learning about yourself and the way you are moving through life, and how that motion might be enriched.

WHAT IS HEALTH COMPETENCE?

The *pathways* of health competence are: 1) health accounting and information gathering; 2) emotional-spiritual health; 3) eating, moving, and habits; 4) illness and problem care (including working with doctors and the system).

For traveling each pathway, a number of *approaches* and *skills* are needed. Here are a few examples. In the health accounting and information gathering pathway, you will need to do such varied tasks as taking your own blood pressure and constructing chart(s) to depict your progress with medical problems. The emotional-spiritual health pathway will ask you (among other things) to learn about the importance of delayed gratification and to practice listening more intently to other people. Eating, moving, and habits are facilitated by learning about your "target zone" for exercise pulse rate and factors affecting appetite. The skills involved in working with your doctor include assertiveness and learning how to clearly tell your medical (or health) story. See Table 1-1 for further examples.

HOW DO YOU BECOME HEALTH COMPETENT?

To become health competent you have to do some things. First, you will need to dust out some of the cobwebs in your attitude closet. You'll have to change your frame of mind and revise your personal health beliefs. You will become increasingly aware that you are the most important and powerful influence on your individual health and medical affairs, and that effective *use* of your own strengths, assets, and knowledge will truly further your health. Your physician is an important and useful person for your health but not omnipotent. Accept that your health is in *your* hands; you must acknowledge ownership.

Then you will need to learn how to use the health competence pathways. It is not necessary for you to follow all of them at once, but steady and disciplined attention to one or more of them (and gradually others) will be necessary. Table 1-1 lists those pathways and tells what they will help you do.

tality and health. She used a number of pathways to do that.

MRS. SCHULTZ

Mildred Schultz was 61 when she first came to Clem's practice. After her initial appraisal, it was clear that she was more than 40 pounds above optimum weight, had poorly controlled diabetes, an uncertain degree of heart disease, and arthritis. She was taking seven different prescription drugs a day! She seemed "apparently dependent on her numerous medications, anxious, mistrusting, and at times downright hostile."

During her first few visits to the center,

TABLE 1–1.

Health Competence Pathway	What It Will Help You Do (some examples)
health accounting and basic skills (Part II)	• periodic personal health assessments on which plans for improving health can be based • maintain your personal health record
emotional-spiritual health (Part III)	• learning and practicing principles of emotional health and personal support • understanding yourself • relating effectively to others • developing and maintaining a support system
eating, moving, and habits (Part IV)	• differentiate categories of exercise • start and maintain an aerobic program • utilize established nutritional principles • manage weight • learn what the unhealthy habits are and a process for changing them
illness and problem care (Part V)	• become more capable of defining and caring for your own medical problems, both alone and in partnership with your physician

Finally, negotiating each pathway requires you to use a number of skills and approaches. Some of them you may know already; others you will need to acquire or apply differently than you do now. Most of the skills are not complicated to learn, but they do require diligence and discipline in their application.

The following story is about an elderly woman who changed herself from a sick, depressed, and dying person to one of vi-

Mrs. Schultz was alternately demanding and passive, sometimes crying. Her former physician had retired and she only came initially to have her prescriptions filled. This was done with the understanding that she would engage in the full health care process. As part of that process she had to decide which of her problems to work on first. She was paralyzed when faced with an actual choice but finally decided to work on her weight. Clem's colleague, Rosemary, began working with Mrs. Schultz to analyze her eating habits and help her learn some basic nutrition and food planning. This, of course, involved making choices again. And try as she might, Mrs. Schultz couldn't get Rosemary to make those choices for her. She learned that she herself could make mistakes, and the world wouldn't end! To facilitate her weight loss, she decided to exercise. She walked, a block a day at first, then gradually increased until after a month, she was walking two miles a day. Then she asked to come into the office and ride the stationary bicycle twice a week also. She lived alone, had no close-by relatives or friends, and probably was as much interested in the company as the exercise. She got increasing amounts of both.

Within eight months Mrs. Schultz was down to her optimum weight, eating healthy food, riding the bike twice a week (five "miles" each time), and walking two to four miles every day. Her diabetes was completely controlled (at this point none of the tests even revealed that she was a diabetic), and her joints were more mobile, infrequently painful, and caused her no significant limitation of activity. *Of the original seven medications she was taking only one*, digitalis for her heart. Clem was not even sure she needed that. Her personality had changed from that of a depressed, passive-aggressive aging lady, to a joyful, outgoing, confident person. She had, from the day of the first diet discussion, participated in all of the decisions about her care and had for the last three to four months made practically all of them on her own and then reported them to Clem and Rosemary. This had included stopping four of her medicines. Each time she did this she came to the office and used the reference books to learn about the medication, such as what it was supposed to be for and its side effects. Then she talked to Clem or Rosemary, and on the basis of all this information made her decisions. She had entered a collaborative partnership and was responsible for herself and her medical care. She felt she was, acted like she was, and was, indeed, in control!

This book is best used by initially reading and working through the exercises in Part II. Thereafter, one can either proceed with the remaining pages in order or move around from chapter to chapter depending on your interests or needs at a particular time. I believe the principles expressed are sound ones that will stand the test of time (or have already stood the test of time). When this is not the case, I will not hesitate to point that out. This book of *Personal Health Competence* can be a companion and assistant to you for a long time to come.

Written to facilitate your attainment of basic personal health competence, this book does not just provide answers. It also will help you ask the right questions— education begins when the right questions are asked. It is not full of solutions, but rather guides you through the process of finding your own solutions. And it is not a crusading, overly cheerful book. It is positive and hopeful, while acknowledging that doing these things is difficult, that there are pitfalls, and that some people may progress slowly, which doesn't mean they're bad or crazy or weak! Above all, being health competent is fun. Don't forget that greater enjoyment of yourself and others is a high priority goal.

Some years ago, almost nineteen hundred to be exact, Plutarch wrote:

Each person ought neither to be unacquainted with the peculiarities of his own pulse (for there are many individual diversities), nor ignorant of any idiosyncrasy which his body has in regard to temperature and dryness, and what things in actual practice have proved to be beneficial or detrimental to it. For the man has no perception regarding himself, and is but a blind and deaf tenant in his own body, who gets his knowledge of these matters from another, and must inquire of his physician whether his health is better in summer or winter, whether he can more easily tolerate liquid or solid foods, and whether his pulse is naturally fast or slow. For it is useful and easy for us to know things of this sort, since we have daily experience and association with them.

I believe he was talking about Personal Health Competence!

Part **II**

THE PATHWAY OF HEALTH ACCOUNTING AND INFORMATION GATHERING

BECOMING competent involves learning where you are, including your strengths and weaknesses, deciding where you are going, and then acquiring the skills you need to get you there. Add some frills and that's what Part II is all about.

By doing your own health appraisal (Chapter 2) you will learn what your health status is now (where you are) and increase awareness about your strengths and weaknesses, although all of them may not become apparent until you have read further in the book. Chapter 3 outlines a way of formulating the Personal Health Guide. This process begins by making Problems Lists which are summaries of your appraisal. Then it continues by developing plans for meeting those problems (where you are going), prioritizing the plans, and developing a schedule for reaching your health goals by implementing the high priority plans (how you will get there).

Chapter 4 teaches one excellent way of keeping a Self-Health Record. Keeping a written record is not part of gaining competence in all endeavors, but the potential complexity of your health makes record keeping an essential skill of Personal Health Competence. Although doctors and hospitals all keep individual patient records, you need something which is unified and all in one place. A written record is strongly advised.

The last chapter in this section, "Gathering and Describing Health Information," will introduce you to further skills which are basic to all parts of Personal Health Competence. They will enhance and enable whatever you decide to do to improve your health and well-being.

These chapters contain a lot of material. It is placed early in the book because these tools are the foundation of a vigorous program for Personal Health Competence. It is a good idea to do the assessment and the plan as soon as possible, as they provide the initial direction and energy for your personal program of health. Other than that, you do not have to learn all this material before you proceed. In fact, most of these skills will be better and more profitably mastered as your personal program progresses.

2

Taking Your Inventory of Health, Well-Being, and Problems

WHAT are your long-term goals for personal health? What changes do you wish to make from your present health status? How will you engineer those changes? These questions serve as a starting point for enhancing Personal Health Competence. Until you know where you are, how can you know or move to where you would like to be? And that's the purpose of this chapter: to help determine your starting point.

The inventory you experience in this chapter will give you a comprehensive overview of where you are healthwise — it is holistic. Although not the kind which predicts the number of years you might add to your life if you give up smoking or control your blood pressure (such predictions are only average estimates anyway), it will give you a broad picture and enough specific information to make good decisions and plan (Chapter 3).

This inventory is divided into five major parts. Each part will touch on physical, intellectual, and emotional-spiritual health. Some questions will explore only one of these areas, others more than one.

Certain questions require factual answers ("List your major medical problems in the past"). Others will stimulate you to explore your health beliefs and personal values and commit yourself to certain goals and courses of action ("What are your health goals?"). Some questions will tell you how to improve your well-being if you choose to do so.

Part A clarifies your health goals and resources, and charts a course toward the goals. Part B provides a picture of your past and present medical/health problems. Part C identifies medical and health problems of potential importance to you in the future (your hidden health problems). Part D charts the habits and lifestyle elements which impinge on your health both now and in the future. Finally, Part E emphasizes your personal health assets (the positive side of the ledger).

PART A: YOUR PERSONAL GOALS, RESOURCES, AND COURSE

This group of questions provides a framework for the rest of the inventory. To define your health goals it may be helpful to think in terms of exercise, nutrition, healthy habits (seat belt use, not smoking), emotional-spiritual health and the quality of your relationship(s) with a health provider, then to formulate one or two goals in one or more of those categories. Make them reasonable both in number and time of attainment.

The questions

1. What is (are) your purpose(s) in life?
2. How does your life work toward those purposes? How against?
3. What are your long-term health goals; how do they relate to your purposes in life?
4. When do you expect to reach these health goals?
5. What strategies and practices will you use to reach these goals?
6. How many hours per week are you willing to invest in health at this time?
7. How much money?
8. Do you have family members, good friends, or co-workers who might accompany you on all or some parts of your journey?
9. Are there other resources not already mentioned which could help you reach your goals?
10. What barriers or problems might pre-

vent you from reaching them or slow you down?
11. Which of your personality characteristics will work for or against you in reaching your goals?

Write out your answers on a suitable piece of paper or in a spiral notebook.

A lot of people have never written out their purposes in life. *Doing so can be a health giving experience.* With your overall purpose clearly (or even unclearly) stated, it is possible to see which aspects of your life will help you accomplish those purposes and which will hinder you.

PART B: YOUR PAST AND PRESENT PROBLEMS

List any important health and medical problems, physical or emotional-spiritual, that you have had in the past or have now. You decide what is important, but include any major illness or surgery from the past and anything of definite or possible importance to your present or future health or well-being. Some of the commoner problems are included in the following list. The terms may be used as they appear or modified to better describe the problem. This list is not complete—you may have a number that are not on the list.

frequent colds or upper respiratory infections
high blood pressure
irregular menses
painful menses
vaginal discharge
heavy menses
light menses
painful knee (elbow, wrist, hip, ankle)
muscle spasm (name place)
low back pain
neck pain
cough
headache
chest pain

poor appetite
weight loss
abdominal pain
loose bowel movements
cancer
heart disease
constipation
allergies
overweight
major surgery (type)
frequent bowel movements
bladder infections
kidney infections
skin rash
skin bumps
ulcer
colitis
acne
nervousness
anxiety
fear (name source if known)
smoking
absent from work a lot
drinking too much or too often
worry
not getting along with wife, husband or
    partner
not getting along with children
angry a lot
frustrated a lot
uncertain about life
unhappy
depressed
not sleeping well
irritable
overstressed

In your PHC notebook list any of the above which apply to you and any other important health and medical problems that you have now or have had. For each item in the list include a brief note about important symptoms, physical findings (if you know them), management, treatment, and the names of doctors, hospitals, and other health workers involved.

Including some of your old problems may or may not be important. For exam-

ple, a forearm fracture 10 years ago that healed well leaving no disability does not affect your present health status. Leave it off. But removal of your gall bladder or appendix is important no matter when it occurred. Any abdominal pain you experience must be considered in light of missing or repaired organs. Also, just surgically opening the abdomen can sometimes cause difficulties years later. *If in doubt about a problem, leave it on the list.*

If you are like most people, the list you have just completed will emphasize physical and medical problems and injuries. To be sure that your emotional-spiritual inventory is complete think carefully through an average or representative day at home, school, work. Then, respond to the following questions, recording the answers in your notebook:

1. What kind of "hassles" are common?
2. Is there any pattern to them?
3. Do you have/receive a comfortable and sufficient level of attention, caring, and listening from others?
4. Do you get "out of yourself" each day?
5. Do you have sufficient time for introspection and being alone each day?
6. What do you do to enrich your spirit?

Recall a recent "bad day."

7. In what way(s) was it bad?
8. Is this a repetitive pattern?
9. Did you seek support from friends, colleagues, your God?

And

10. What is your general morale like?
11. Do you laugh and cry?
12. Do you feel lonely, angry, sad?

In his book, *The Road Less Traveled*, Peck emphasizes personal discipline as an essential part of emotional-spiritual health.[1] To further broaden your emo-

1. M.S. Peck, *The Road Less Traveled*. (New York: Touchstone, Siomon & Schuster, 1978).

tional-spiritual inventory here are some questions about discipline which may help identify areas you want to work on.

Responsibility for Self:

1. When you have a misfortune or things don't go quite the way you planned, do you tend to put the "blame" on yourself or others?
2. To what extent do you believe you control the course of your life, as opposed to other people, God, fate, or some force outside of you?
3. When you become ill do you tend to see it as fate, bad luck, coincidence, or as a result of the way you have been living?

Delayed Gratification:

4. If you have a job to be done and a pleasure to be enjoyed, do you, as a rule, do the work before the pleasure? Do you get your homework done before enjoying TV, your housework before going out to lunch?

Openness to challenge:

5. To what extent do you, in the course of daily work and living, look for, seek out, accept, listen to, or tune out the comments of others with respect to your behavior, work abilities, competence, and performance?
6. Do you change behaviors (ways of doing things), opinions, style—often or never? Is your way the right way? Are you embarrassed or angered by having your way challenged?

Dedication to truth:

7. Do you tell outright lies, cheat on your expense accounts, income tax, engage in secret activities which could harm others (like affairs), lie to family and business associates, believe that "little lies are OK" if they "help" people?
8. Are you untruthful about your motives if you think the listener may be offended, shocked, insulted, or angered by the truth? Are you untruthful when you think it will cause less hassle or be less trouble?

Write any comments in relation to the above in your notebook.

Take your list of past and present problems seriously but be realistic. Accept responsibility for them and acknowledge your own part in their initiation and maintenance. This is a prime requisite for health competence. Ask whether they require modification of your *approach* to greater health, understanding they cannot constrain your attainment of greater health. We can all be healthier than we are.

This part of your inventory provides a picture of how things have been and are now with respect to your health and medical affairs. It may also reveal caution signs. Frequent respiratory infections each year during your company's annual change-over period may indicate that you need to find additional ways of handling stress at those times. If you have had accidents more than once during the holiday season, you might consider the relationship of alcohol to your propensity for accidents, or the emotional stress of those times.

PART C: IDENTIFYING YOUR POTENTIAL HEALTH AND MEDICAL PROBLEMS

The concept of potential problems is critical to health and well-being. Identifying potential problems is a mandatory first step in preventing them or lessening their impact. They are identified in four ways: from the family history, from a close look at your living and working environment, from consideration of the problems which most frequently involve people of your own age/sex/race, and from your own habits and life-style. The first three of these are the focus of Inventory Part C. The last is the subject of Part D.

To do your *family history* write down the present age (or age at death) for your father, mother, brothers, and sisters. After their names write any serious medical problems they have had or have now

TABLE 2–1a[4]   Showing the five leading causes of death in the next ten years for individuals 15–70 years old now. Each figure represents the number of deaths per 100,000 people from the designated condition.

White Females

Condition	15	20	25	30	35	40	45	50	55	60	65	70
Motor Vehicle Accidents	197	139	103	90								
Suicide	52	77	91	105	125							
Homicide	40	45	66									
Poisonings	17	17	38									
Leukemia	17											
Vascular Lesions of CNS (Stroke)			20	60	108	174	268	422	699	1,241	2,464	5,079
Cancer of the Breast			31	97	186	342	518	684	807	859	921	1,018
AHD[2](Heart Attack)				54	136	308	624	1,260	2,406	4,307	7,755	13,666
Cirrhosis					101	170	232	284				
Cancer of the Lung						149	249	386	517	501		
Cancer of Large Bowel/Rectum									434	631	900	1,232
Diseases of the Arteries											388	853
TOTAL OF ALL CONDITIONS[3]	590	650	810	1,170	1,809	2,872	4,328	6,567	9,821	14,441	22,448	37,203

TABLE 2–1b[4].

White Males

Condition	Age Group											
	15	20	25	30	35	40	45	50	55	60	65	70
Motor Vehicle Accidents	691	581	403	325	290	275	281					
Suicide	189	250	240	244	250	260						
Homicide	120	164	163	159	148							
Drownings	82	69	62									
Poisonings	59	64										
Other Accidents												
AHD[2] (Heart Attack)			71	254	723	1,629	2,973	5,001	7,809	11,273	15,622	21,374
Cirrhosis				98	200	343	471	580	667			
Cancer of the Lung						348	681	1,188	1,888	2,561	2,998	3,176
Vascular Lesions CNS[1]							299	541	979	1,775	3,218	5,583
Cancer of Large Bowel/Rectum								314	530	814	1,121	1,464
Bronchitis and Emphysema										736	1,152	1,552
TOTAL OF ALL CONDITIONS[3]	1,760	1,765	1,771	2,148	3,200	5,237	8,298	13,267	20,694	30,483	43,950	63,436

TABLE 2-1c[4].

Black Females

Condition	Age Group											
	15	20	25	30	35	40	45	50	55	60	65	70
Homicide	247	313	300	288	259	196						
Motor Vehicle Accidents	105	112	106									
Pregnancy and Abortion	38											
Poisonings	38	51										
Suicide	37	48										
Vascular Lesions CNS[1]		47	96	187	358	597	893	1,348	2,007	3,032	5,210	7,485
Cirrhosis			122	241	351	468	486	458				
AHD[2](Heart Attack)			76	200	490	1,061	1,834	3,042	4,697	6,782	11,110	15,157
Cancer of the Breast				136	251	404	584	703	730	748	826	
Cancer of the Lung							311	421	487			
Cancer of Large Bowel/Rectum									491	638	946	1,133
Hypertensive Heart Disease										512	800	1,016
Diseases of the Arteries												1,082
TOTAL OF ALL CONDITIONS[3]	1,070	1,472	1,949	2,892	4,337	6,432	9,075	12,752	17,320	22,764	35,440	47,528

TABLE 2-1d[4].

Black Males

Condition	Age Group											
	15	20	25	30	35	40	45	50	55	60	65	70
Homicide	1,038	1,596	1,617	1,501	1,340	1,110	987	806				
Motor Vehicle Accidents	422	521	472	431	422							
Drownings	185	140										
Suicide	123	216	223									
Poisonings	80	138										
Cirrhosis			215	448	651	834	919	878	783			
AHD[2] (Heart Attack)			159	415	977	2,034	3,476	5,332	7,608	10,138	14,229	18,323
Vascular Lesions CNS[1]				197		677	1,029	1,583	2,400	3,514	5,367	7,382
Cancer of the Lung						607	1,183	1,893	2,437	2,709	2,958	2,834
Pneumonia									683	856	1,165	1,677
Cancer of Prostate										984	1,820	2,671
TOTAL OF ALL CONDITIONS[3]	2,851	4,252	4,948	6,034	7,972	10,993	15,259	21,154	28,231	35,914	49,088	63,564

1. CNS = Central Nervous System (brain and spinal cord).
2. AHD = Arteriosclerotic Heart Disease.
3. Only the first five conditions in each age group are listed, hence the numbers in the last horizontal line are more than the total of the column of figures above them.
4. These tables were compiled from data found in Geller, H., Steele, G. 1974 Probability Tables of Dying in the next 10 years from specific causes (Indianapolis, IN: Methodist Hospital, 1974).

(like heart attacks, high blood pressure, cancer, allergies).

In addition to the problems you have just listed, add others that you know "run" in the family. Try and identify "tendencies," problems which seem to have recurred in different members or generations of the family. Don't put down things that have occurred once, unless you know they are often inherited.

Next is *the environment*. Think about your home, school, workplace. Identify any obvious or potential hazards to your health (poisons, polluted air, emotional manipulation, hyperstress). Remember to think in terms of both emotional-spiritual health and physical health, e.g., an abusive alcoholic family member might be a threat to both physical and emotional health.

Now look at Tables 2-1a through 2-1d. By finding your age group, sex, and race, you can find the names of those problems which might seriously jeopardize your health in the next five years. Write them down on the left side of a new page in your notebook.

For example, as a 55-year old white male, the greatest threats to me are coronary artery disease (heart attack), cancer of the lung, and circulatory problems in the brain (mainly strokes). Respiratory disease, skin disease, and digestive disorders are less likely trouble areas. For Frank (black, male, 27), the three top threats are homicide, auto accident, and suicide.

In Table 2-2 each of the "threats to life" are listed again. The second column gives the health factors which increase your risk for the corresponding condition. Many of them are controllable. By working on these factors, you can probably reduce your chances of succumbing to one or more of your big five. For example, smoking cigarettes not only increases the odds that you will get cancer of the lung, it also increases the odds of a heart attack and

the pesky, common upper respiratory infection. For each of your three or four greatest threats note the factor or factors which increase your risk.

Parts C and D begin to sketch out the future. Each section may show you where certain risks are, and the steps you must take to reduce them. In providing this kind of information, these sections are more important than the others. Using the metaphor of a journey by ship, Parts C and D of the inventory reveal the dangerous currents, the hidden reefs, and the potential storms of your voyage. You can take steps to reduce the impact of many of them.

PART D: POTENTIAL PROBLEMS (HABITS AND LIFE-STYLE)

This section of the inventory (Table 2-3) is a survey of your habits and life-style. It is the last step in identifying potential or hidden problems. It asks about so-called health practices. For some, the relationship to your health is pretty obvious (like smoking). For others, it may not be clear until you have read further in the book. (An asterisk following an item indicates further explanation in the footnotes at the end of the survey.)

PART E: STRENGTHS AND ASSETS

Now it is critical to tabulate personal strengths and assets; it can be discouraging to only list problems. Positive attributes can be real assets in attaining better health. *It is important not to forget this.* Think of the physical, intellectual, and emotional-spiritual strengths which are or can be employed in your work and personal life. Also list supportive resources like friends, tight-knit family, or financial security. Greg, for example, wrote down: a family history of long life, a sharp mind, skill at working harmoni- *(continued on p. 31)*

Table 2–2.

Threat to Life	Factors Which Increase Risk
Arteriosclerotic Heart Disease (Heart Attack)	high-fat diet, untreated high blood pressure, smoking, little exercise
Bronchitis and Emphysema	smoking, environmental pollution
Cancer of the Large Bowel and Rectum	high-fat diet
Cancer of the Lung	smoking, environmental pollution
Cirrhosis	excess use of alcohol
Diseases of the Arteries	untreated high blood pressure, high-fat diet
Drownings	not learning to swim, not following water safety rules
Homicide	poverty and need, handguns, gang warfares, suppression and repression of anger, prison conditions, alcohol and drug abuse
Hypertensive Heart Disease (due to high blood pressure)	untreated high blood pressure; high salt intake; unresolved stress and tension
Motor Vehicle Accidents	not wearing seat belts, drinking and driving, exceeding speed limit, unbelted tires, poor brakes
Pneumonia	smoking, poverty, alcohol and drug abuse, malnutrition
Poisonings	careless use and storage of toxic materials and medicines
Suicide	isolation, depression, fear of and or inability to get psychiatric care, alcohol and drug abuse
Vascular Lesions of the Central Nervous System (Stroke)	high-fat diet, untreated high blood pressure, insufficient exercise

TABLE 2–3   Habit & Life-style Questionnaire.

A. Eating Habits

	Always	Mostly	Sometimes	Never
1. I eat a variety of foods, such as fruits and vegetables, whole grain breads and cereals, lean meats, dairy products, dry peas and beans, and nuts and seeds.	____	____	____	____
2. I limit the amount of fat, saturated fat, and cholesterol I eat (including fat on meats, eggs, butter, cream, shortenings), and organ meats such as liver.	____	____	____	____
3. I limit the amount of salt I eat by cooking with only small amounts, not adding salt at the table, and avoiding salty snacks.	____	____	____	____
4. I avoid eating too much sugar (especially frequent snacks of sticky candy or soft drinks).	____	____	____	____
5. I eat breakfast.*	____	____	____	____
6. I add unprocessed bran to my food to provide roughage.†	____	____	____	____
7. I drink less than 3 cups of coffee or tea a day (herbal teas excepted).*†	____	____	____	____
8. I try to eat only unprocessed foods.	____	____	____	____

B. Safety Habits

	Always	Mostly	Sometimes	Never
1. I wear a shoulder/lap belt while riding in a car.*†	————	————	————	————
2. I avoid driving while under the influence of alcohol and other drugs.	————	————	————	————
3. I obey traffic rules and the speed limit when driving.	————	————	————	————
4. I am careful when using potentially harmful products or substances (such as household cleaners, poisons, and electrical devices).*	————	————	————	————
5. I avoid smoking in bed.	————	————	————	————
6. I minimize my exposure to sprays, chemical fumes, or exhaust gases.*†	————	————	————	————
7. I avoid extremely noisy areas (or wear protective ear plugs).†	————	————	————	————
8. I frequently inspect my automobile tires, lights, etc., and have my car serviced regularly.†	————	————	————	————
9. I have disc brakes on my car.*†	Yes			No
10. I drive on belted radial tires.*†	Yes			No
11. I have a dry chemical fire extinguisher in my kitchen and at least one other elsewhere in my living quarters. (For a very small apartment, kitchen extinguisher is adequate.)†	Yes			No

C. Fitness, Exercise, and Activity*

	Almost Always	Sometimes	Almost Never
1. I maintain a desired weight, avoiding overweight and underweight.	————	————	————
2. I do vigorous exercise for 25–30 minutes at least 3 times a week (examples include running, swimming, brisk walking).	————	————	————
3. I do exercise that enhances my muscle tone for 15–30 minutes at least 3 times a week (examples include yoga and calisthenics).	————	————	————
4. I use part of my leisure time participating in individual, family, or team activities that increase my level of fitness (such as gardening, bowling, golf, and baseball).	————	————	————
5. I do yoga or some form of stretching/limbering exercise for 15 to 20 minutes at least 3 times per week.†	————	————	————

† Questions taken from *Wellness Inventory*, used with permission, copyright 1975, 1981, John W. Travis, M.D., Wellness Associates, Box 5433, Mill Valley, CA 94942. Abridged from the *Wellness Workbook*, Ryan & Travis, Ten Speed Press, 1981.

* See Footnotes to Habit and Life-style Questionnaire, p. 30.

D. Relaxation, Stress

1. I have a job or do other work that I enjoy.	Yes	No	Not Sure
2. I find it easy to relax and express my feelings freely and do so.	Daily	Sometimes	Rarely
3. I recognize early, and prepare for, events or situations likely to be stressful for me.*	Yes	No	Sometimes
4. I have close friends, relatives, or others whom I can talk to about personal matters and call on for help when needed.	Yes	No	Sometimes
5. I participate in group activities (such as church and community organizations) or hobbies that I enjoy.	Yes	No	Sometimes
6. I sleep 7 or more hours per night.	Yes	No	Sometimes
7. I am *always* on the go.*	Yes	No	Sometimes
8. I have a sense of time urgency/impatience.*	Yes	No	Sometimes
9. I feel tired and rundown.	Yes	No	Sometimes
10. I bite or pick at my nails.	Yes	No	Sometimes

E. Use of Alcohol and Drugs

	Always	Mostly	Sometimes	Never
1. I avoid drinking alcoholic beverages *or* I drink no more than 1 or 2 drinks a day.*	_____	_____	_____	_____
2. I avoid using alcohol or other drugs (especially illegal drugs) as a way of handling stressful situations or the problems in my life.*	_____	_____	_____	_____
3. I am careful not to drink alcohol when taking certain medicines (for example, medicine for sleeping, pain, colds, and allergies), or when pregnant.*	_____	_____	_____	_____
4. I read and follow the label directions when using prescribed and over-the-counter drugs.	_____	_____	_____	_____
5. I use "street" drugs.	Daily	Occasionally	Rarely	Never
6. I use prescribed tranquilizers or mood altering drugs.	Daily	Occasionally	Rarely	Never
7. I rarely take medicine of any kind.	Yes			No

F. Personal Health

	Yes	No
1. I regularly use dental floss and a soft toothbrush.*†	_____	_____
WOMEN		
2. I check my breasts for unusual lumps once a month.†	_____	_____
3. I have a pap test annually.†	_____	_____
MEN		
4. If uncircumcised, I am aware of the special need for regular cleansing under my foreskin.†	_____	_____
5. If over 45, I have my prostate checked annually. I examine my testes every six months for lumps.†	_____	_____

G. Smoking Habits

	Yes	No
1. I don't smoke at all.†	_____	_____
2. I avoid smoking cigarettes.	_____	_____
3. If you don't smoke now, how long has it been? _____		
4. I smoke less than one pack of cigarettes or equivalent cigars or pipes per week.†	_____	_____
5. I smoke _____ cigarettes/pipes/cigars a day.		
6. I have smoked this much (question 5) or more for _____ years.		

H. Emotional-Spiritual Health*

Check each item that you think describes your own state of mind and/or behavior.†

1. ____ Rather than worrying, I can temporarily shelve my problems and enjoy myself at times when I can do nothing about solving them immediately.
2. ____ I am content with my sexual life.
3. ____ I am frequently happy.
4. ____ I think it is OK to feel angry, afraid, joyful, or sad.
5. ____ I do not deny my anger, fear, joy or sadness, but instead find constructive ways to express these feelings most of the time.
6. ____ I am able to say "no" to people without feeling guilty.
7. ____ It is easy for me to laugh.
8. ____ I like getting compliments and recognition from other people.
9. ____ I feel OK about crying and allow myself to do so.
10. ____ I listen to and think about constructive criticism rather than react defensively.
11. ____ I would seek help from friends and professional counselors if needed.
12. ____ It is easy for me to give other people sincere compliments and recognition.
13. ____ I make an attempt to know my neighbors and be on good terms with them.
14. ____ If I saw a crime being committed, I would call the police.
15. ____ If I saw a broken bottle lying in the road or on the sidewalk, I would remove it.
16. ____ If I saw a car with faulty lights, leaking gasoline, or another dangerous condition, I would attempt to inform the driver.
17. ____ I have sought information on parenting and raising children.
18. ____ I frequently touch or hold my children.
19. ____ I respect my child as an evolving, growing being.
20. ____ I am aware of changes in my physical or mental state, and seek professional advice about any which seem unusual.
21. ____ I enjoy spending some time without planned or structured activities.
22. ____ I enjoy touching other people.
23. ____ I have at least five close friends.
24. ____ At times I like to be alone.
25. ____ I like myself and look forward to the future.
26. ____ I look forward to living to be at least 75.
27. ____ I find it easy to express concern, love, and warmth to those I care about.
28. ____ I consider myself a spiritually active person.*

† Questions 1–27 in part taken from *Wellness Inventory*, used with permission, copyright 1975, 1981, John W. Travis, M.D., Wellness Associates, Box 5433, Mill Valley, CA 94942. Abridged from the *Wellness Workbook*, Ryan & Travis, Ten Speed Press, 1981.

* See Footnotes to Habit and Life-style Questionnaire, p. 30.

For the next series of questions check the response which most nearly describes your behavior.

	Always	Mostly	Sometimes	Never
29. My communication with others is open, honest, and clear.				
30. I give and receive affection.				
31. I have feelings of anger and hostility.				
32. I am a positive thinker.				
33. I am anxious and worry.				
34. I am depressed.				
35. I have good relationships with those around me.				
36. I have communion with some power I regard as greater than myself.				
37. I engage in activities which I believe enrich my spirit.				
38. I would say that I am honest.				

I. Measurements

1. My blood pressure is usually: (check one upper and one lower number)
   100   110   120   130   140   150   160   more than 160
   _____
   60   70   80   90   100   110   120   more than 120

2. My weight is: _____.*

3. My serum or plasma cholesterol is: (check nearest number)*
   100   125   150   175   200   225   250   275   300   more than 300

† Questions taken from *Wellness Inventory*, used with permission, copyright 1975, 1981, John W. Travis, M.D., Wellness Associates, Box 5433, Mill Valley, CA 94942. Abridged from the *Wellness Workbook*, Ryan & Travis, Ten Speed Press, 1981.

FOOTNOTES TO HABIT AND LIFE-STYLE QUESTIONNAIRE

A	5	At least one major study shows that people who regularly eat breakfast are healthier than those who don't.
A	7	Caffeine is a mood altering substance to which people can become habituated. Caffeine accelerates heart rate, increases sweating (in some people), and can increase blood pressure and the tendency to muscle spasm in some people.
B	1	Shoulder/lap belts provide much higher margins of safety than lap belts alone.
B	4 &6	Exposure to any strong chemicals or toxic substances should be avoided as much as possible. While local injury (such as a chemical burn or respiratory tract irritation) is of significant concern, an even greater threat is the possibility that cancer and degenerative diseases may be caused or accelerated by a variety of presently unknown agents.
B	9	Disk brakes do a better job than drum breaks.
B	10	Radial tires provide better braking and better gas mileage.
C		Exercise is important for cardiovascular conditioning, flexibility, and increasing muscular strength and definition. Part IV covers the issues raised by these questions in some detail.
D	3	One way to reduce dysfunctional stress is to adequately prepare for situations known to be stressful to you.
D	7 &8	Being constantly on the go and the sense of time urgency and impatience are characteristics of the Type A personality which is more prone to heart attack.
E	1	The exact level of alcohol consumption that spells trouble differs a lot between individuals. Habitual daily consumption of any amount is one danger signal of alcoholism. Getting into trouble (any kind) while drinking is another.
E	2	This pattern is one that may signal addiction or be an avenue to addiction.

E	3	Many medications contain substances which potentiate or confuse the effects of alcohol in dangerous ways.
F	1	Regular flossing and brushing not only reduce the incidence of cavities but help prevent plaque (tartar) accumulation. Plaque in turn causes gum disease which is the main cause of tooth loss in mid- and late-adult life.
G		A yes for one is healthiest. Pipes and cigars are (generally) more healthy than cigarettes because they usually are not inhaled. Oral cancer as a result of pipe smoking is not uncommon. A year after you stop smoking entirely your chances of avoiding lung cancer have greatly improved, but do not become normal until ten years later.
H		Statements 1–28 in this section are worded positively. Each of these things that you do on some regular basis is healthy. Part III (The Pathway of Emotional-Spiritual Health) discusses many of these items in more detail. Repression of emotions is not healthy. Constructive (or non-destructive) expression is desirable but at times hard to attain. When the latter is frequently true, it is good to get a therapist or counselor who can help the individual relearn emotional awareness and healthy expression. The use of emotions to control and manipulate others is not healthy.
H	28	In responding to items 28, 36, and 37, use your own definition of "spiritual."
I	1	In general, the lower one's regular blood pressure is, the better it is for long-term health. The generally expected "normal" pressure for the U.S. is 130/80 or less, but optimal blood pressure for long-term health is more like 100/60.
II	2	See Chapter 14 for a discussion of optimal weight (or body fat).
I	3	The lower your total serum or plasma cholesterol, the better (i.e., the less your risk of heart disease). Everyone should strive for cholesterol of 180 or less.

ously with people, high energy, self-esteem, and confidence. I cannot put the first one on my list but the rest also apply to me. In addition, I am in good aerobic condition, financially secure, like my work, and have a group of loyal and loving friends and family.

Begin by writing down whatever comes to mind. Then look through the earlier parts of this appraisal. Various items will remind you of other strengths. Then use the following checklist to facilitate the sometimes difficult task of identifying your own strengths and assets. *It is by no means comprehensive.* If any of these items reflect an asset, put it down, but don't confine your list to the items found here. Individuals have their own idiosyncracies and some of those are strengths, even though they might not be considered as such by others.

- devotion to a hobby
- steadfast church or club affiliation
- athletically fit
- good eyesight
- no serious illness
- ability to communicate
- openness in communication
- willing to listen to criticism
- good listener in general
- effective speaker
- financially secure
- cohesive family group
- close friend(s)
- work well with people
- self-confidence
- self-esteem
- enjoy work
- good relationship with partner or spouse
- generally receptive to new ideas
- able to hear other points of view
- inquisitive mind
- handy around the house
- good relationship with boss
- laugh a lot
- good sense of humor
- committed to being good parent
- careful with money
- know and follow good nutritional principles
- believe in God (or some higher power)
- honesty
- solve problems well
- sensitive to the needs of others
- own house
- patience
- sexually happy
- get joy out of life

The section on strengths and attributes completes your personal health appraisal. To the extent you have responded to the various questions and their underlying significance, you have a meaningful assessment. It will serve as a strong foundation for building a program of Health Competence. The next step in that program is to write a Personal Health Guide. The next chapter will help you do that.

RESOURCES CHAPTER 2

Ryan, R.S. and Travis, J.W. *Wellness Workbook* (see General Resources).

3

Your Personal Health Guide

YOUR Personal Health Guide is a blueprint for health and well-being. It evolves from the inventory in the last chapter. If you have only partially completed that inventory, your plan will be correspondingly incomplete, but useful, nevertheless. Developing a coherent and useful plan for health and well-being from your inventory is best done with an orderly approach. This approach is part of Personal Health Competence.

HEALTH GOALS, PAST AND PRESENT PROBLEMS

Using a piece of paper ruled and labeled like Figure 3-1, list your health goals in the top area (from item 3 in Part I of your appraisal — "What are your long term health goals . . . etc."). Next transfer your list of past and present problems to the left upper box from Part II of your inventory.

YOUR POTENTIAL PROBLEMS

The list of potential problems is started by listing the five leading causes of death in your age group (refer to your appraisal). Follow this with any items from your family history (again refer to your appraisal) that represent increased risk for you. If you are not sure about certain ones, look them up in the *Merck Manual*,[1] *Better Homes & Gardens New Family Medical Guide*,[2] or a medical text-

1. D.N. Holvey, ed., *The Merck Manual of Diagnosis and Therapy* (Rahway, NJ: Merck Sharp and Dohme Research Laboratories, 1982).
2. E. Kiester, Jr., ed., Better Homes and Gardens New Family Medical Guide (Des Moines, Iowa: Better Homes and Gardens Books, 1982).

FIGURE 3–1   Your Health Planning Guide.

Health Goals	
Past and Present Problems	*Potential Problems*
Plan	*Plan*
Strengths and Resources	

book at the library. Next list any hazards in the home and environment which might affect your health (see your appraisal). Ask the county health department for help if you're not sure. Then look carefully through your habit and life-style questionnaire and add to the potential problem list any items that suggest changes that could improve your health. They must seem important to you with respect to your health, or be items that you have been told threaten your health. Some are straightforward, like smoking, not wearing seat belts, lack of exercise. Others are more complicated. For example, if you think you drive safely

after three drinks, but your oldest daughter worries about it, the honest choice is to put it down, perhaps indicating that someone else thinks it's a problem but you don't. Put down all the items you want to whether or not you think you might be doing something about them in the near future.

Should you list a habit and life-style item separately when it is related to a problem or potential problem already on one of the two lists? For example, if you are a smoker and have already listed coronary disease (heart attack) as a potential problem, should smoking be listed as a problem as well? When in doubt, do so. In the example given, there would be no doubt — smoking is a problem in and of itself as well as a risk factor for coronary artery disease.

THE PLANNING LISTS

You have now completed the two upper problem boxes with an outline of your past and present problems (on the left) and your potential future problems (on the right).

In the two lower boxes you will outline plans for managing present problems (on the left) and plans for maintaining health and increasing well-being (on the right) for the next five years. Those items in the left-hand planning box may have to be instituted immediately (if, indeed, they are not already being done) in order to properly manage existing conditions and prevent their recurrence.

Develop plan items by listing one or more strategies that might be used to manage or prevent each item in the problem list above it. Put down logical things *whether or not* you think you will ever carry them out. If you smoke cigarettes and agree that they are a risk to your health, put down "stop smoking" even though, right now, that seems impossible to you.

Some strategies will relate to more than one problem on your list. If so, this will be a factor to consider when you prioritize the items in the plan. Obviously "Start using seat belts 100%" is a strategy that applies specifically to one problem. "Begin regular program of aerobic exercise," however, might apply to several potential problems: coronary artery disease, smoking, overweight, or depression (as well as others). Look for two or more items on your problem list that might benefit from the same strategy.

Write plan items for the emotional, social, and work problems as well as for the "physical" ones. This may be where you need to start.

Greg's Health Planning Guide is represented in Figure 3–2. His achilles tendon and knee cartilage both appear to be well now, so as a plan for these he simply wrote "continue stretching" (Plan I, item 5). He began psychotherapy some months ago. It has been helpful with items 3, 4, 5, and 9 (under Past and Present Problems) — thus, "Continue psychotherapy" was another listing in his plan. For item 7, in Past and Present Problems, the strategy he listed was "Try and discontinue allopurinol and control gout through diet" (Plan I, item 2). "Reduce pipe smoking to one/day" (Plan I, item 3) obviously pertains to problem 8 and "Gradual Weight Reduction" (Plan I, item 6) to problem 6. When he got to problem 9 he thought awhile. He realized that although the therapy has been helpful for the relationships with his children, other emotional issues had gotten priority. He had heard friends talk about attending a parenting workshop and decided to put that down as an additional strategy (Plan I, item 4).

Then he turned to his *potential problems* and made the planning list you see there. He recognized that weight control and less smoking from the Plan I list applied to Potential Problem 1. He had listed "Become aerobically conditioned" as a health goal (it is not reflected directly on either problem list). An exercise program will also apply to Potential Problems 1 and 5, so he listed that. He already uses seat belts, but occasionally drives after drinking. So for items 2, 3, and 7 he lists "Reduce alcohol intake to 1 or 2 drinks daily." He has not ever been suicidal and feels that his therapy covers Potential Problem number 4. "Reducing commitments at work" is a strategy that will help him with both Potential Problems 5 and 6 (and 5 in his other list). "Publish two papers in the next year" is

FIGURE 3–2   Greg's Health Planning Guide.

Health Goals

1. Lose fifteen pounds
2. Become aerobically conditioned
3. Stop smoking
4. Control gout — less than 1 attack/year
5. Have loving non-manipulative relationship with 3 children
6. Committed long-term relationship with a woman

Past and Present Problems	*Potential Problems*
1. Ruptured achilles tendon (left) March '81	1. Coronary artery disease
2. Torn knee cartilage (right) 4/79	2. Motor vehicle accident
3. Separation and divorce, '82	3. Cirrhosis of liver
4. Custody "fight" for children	4. Suicide
5. Becoming a single parent	5. Sequelae of stress at work
6. Overweight 15 pounds	6. Need to publish
7. Gout since '81	7. 4–5 drinks/day
8. Pipe smoking	8. High fat intake
9. Tendency to be manipulative with children	

Plan I	*Plan II*
1. Continue psychotherapy — 3, 4, 5, 9	1. Begin aerobic exercise program — 1, 4, 5 (also present problem 6)
2. Try and discontinue allopurinol and control gout through diet — 7	2. Reduce alcohol to 1–2 drinks/day — 7 (also potential problem 3)
3. Reduce pipe smoking to one pipe/day (also — 8, Potential Problem 1)	3. Reduce commitments at work — 5, 6
4. Take a parenting workshop — 9	4. Write two papers in next year — 6
5. Continue stretching — 1, 2	5. Diet changes phasing into fewer calories, less fat, low purines — 1, 8 (also potential problem 6 and goal 1)
6. Gradual weight reduction	

Strengths and Resources

Greg's direct strategy to handle 6. Finally, he wrote a plan item that describes in general terms how he will alter his diet. This applies to problem 6 in the left list and problems 1 and 8 on the right.

PERSONAL STRENGTHS AND RESOURCES

Do not try to prioritize the steps in your plan or set dates for implementation yet. First, go to the bottom box in the chart and list your strengths and resources. Take them directly from the list you made during your appraisal as well as from the answers to items 7, 8, and 9 in Part I of the appraisal.

PRIORITIZING YOUR PLAN

You have constructed a list of strategies from which you will finalize your plan. Now it is time to prioritize the items in your plan and then develop a reasonable time schedule for implementing the top priority group.

Prioritizing is a difficult and important job. Here are some steps that will help.

1. Mark those items that will impact on two (one check) or more (two checks) of the problems in your list.
2. Place a different kind of mark beside those strategies (activities) you would

like to try — the ones that are interesting and exciting to you.

3. Mark with another symbol those steps that look particularly difficult to you at the present time.

4. Circle those for which there are good resources and support systems available. (If you live close to a high school athletic field and can use their track, that's a good resource for an exercise program.) If your employer has started a health program that includes a stop smoking group, that's a good resource. If there are steps that cost money, then money is a resource that must be considered.

5. Then ask yourself, "What is my thinking about this strategy? What are my fears, questions, doubts, and enthusiasms?"

At this point, it is advisable to review your health goals. Are they measurable? Can they be achieved and definite progress measured in a few months time? "Lose ten pounds in the next three months" is much more helpful than "Lose some weight in the next few months." Be as specific as possible in creating your goals.

Now, "sit with" your planning list and your list of strengths and resources for a few days. Look at it occasionally, paying particular attention to whether the decisions you made in 1-4 above still feel correct to you. If not, change them to correspond with your new feelings. After a week during which you have looked at it a few times (first thing in the morning or last at night are good times), set aside an hour when you won't be interrupted (remember, this is your health plan) and prioritize each of the plan items as 1 (highest priority), 2, or 3. Number all of them. Try and have about equal numbers of items in each group. Finally, take the number 1 group, and write a schedule which covers a two- or

three-year span. Use the format shown in Figure 3-3. You cannot and should not try to do everything at once or too much too fast. Remember that in terms of the length of time it took you to reach the state of health or unhealth that you are in now, a couple of years to begin turning it around is not a long time. You are more likely to have significant success by spacing the plan out than by trying to do it all at once. Once you begin, you may find that certain things will happen sooner anyway.

As a general rule of thumb, it is best to begin with exercise if it's on your list. Meditation, yoga, and more active spirituality are also items on which other strategies can build.

Greg marked his list as shown in Figure 3-4. The single-checked items apply to two of the problems, double checks to more than two. The solid dots mark items that are exciting to Greg, the X's are those that seem particularly difficult. The circles are items for which there are good resources.

Greg then took two weeks during which he glanced at the list almost every day but did not change anything. At the end of that time, he set aside time for himself and developed the following plan.

Begin immediately, have finished (those that can be completed) *or going on* (those that will be on-going) *in one year.*

- complete two research papers — into the hands of the prospective publishers
- take a parenting workshop
- continue psychotherapy
- reduce other work obligations enough so that I can write papers

Begin six months from now (when bulk of work on writing papers should be done)

- aerobic exercise program
- if it has not happened, reduce alcohol intake

FIGURE 3–3   Health Guide: Plan Detail for Accomplishing First Priority Items.

Date _____

I. Begin immediately and have finished (where that is possible, or in progress) one year from now.

_____

_____

_____

_____

_____

_____

II. _____ months from now

_____

_____

_____

_____

_____

III. _____ months from now

_____

_____

_____

_____

_____

IV. _____ years from now

_____

_____

_____

_____

_____

✓✓ 1. Continue psychotherapy
   O 2. Control gout with diet
✗✓ 3. Reduce smoking to one bowl per day
●✓ 4. Take a parenting workshop
    5. Continue stretching

O●✓✓ 1. Begin aerobic exercise program
    ✓ 2. Reduce alcohol to 1–2 drinks/day
    ●✓ 3. Reduce obligations at work
    ✗ 4. Write two papers in next year
O✗✓✓ 5. Change diet to fewer calories, less fat, low purines

FIGURE 3–4 Greg's Marked List.

12–15 months from now

- reassess progress and status at that time
- check priorities; decide whether to continue present plan or alter it
- begin phased dietary changes: start by moving into foods of lower caloric density that are more natural in origin; don't worry about fewer purines (to combat gout) until later, but do check that the changes I am making toward lower caloric density do not increase purine intake.
- reduce pipe smoking to three bowls/day

2 years from now

- reduce pipe smoking to one bowl a day (or stop)
- continue evolution of diet and begin consciously reducing purines as well.

Use a sheet ruled and labeled like the one in Figure 3-3 when you are ready.

In actual practice, Greg did all of the first year as planned. Although he had not counted on it, he was able to stop psychotherapy before the year was out. That gave him a little more leeway and time. Work pressures eased both through his efforts to ease them and because his papers looked good to the boss and were soon accepted for publication. As a result of the second year reassessment, Greg decided to proceed as originally planned. The dietary changes went well, and his weight began to fall at about two pounds a month (he had already lost three pounds in the last half of the first year after beginning to exercise regularly). Reduction in pipe smoking proved to be

a different matter. Now, at the end of the second year, he still smokes it five to nine times a day (the latter when he is under pressure). As we discussed his plan for the third year he was seriously considering joining a stop smoking group to help him quit completely. He is planning to increase his exercise program from three to four or five days a week, and this may help with the pipe.

It may be necessary to break certain steps of the plan into more workable pieces. For example, look at Greg's plan "Begin aerobic exercise program." That is an indistinct statement. It will be more useful to say 1) "Start with walking 20 minutes three times a week; 2) after that time, reevaluate and if OK, start running; 3) learn to take pulse so that I can monitor heart rate during exercise."

Check through your own plan steps to see if they are specific enough to be useful.

MONITORING YOUR HEALTH

Systematic Health Maintenance requires a plan for periodically evaluating your health and medical status. One important component of such a monitoring program is to repeat at three- to five-year intervals the following parts of your self-appraisals: purpose in life, health goals, present problems, main problems for which you are at risk (from Table 1 Chapter 2), Habit & Life-style questionnaire, and strengths and positive attributes.

When restating your health goals, you will find Appendix A to be helpful. It gives health goals for ten distinct developmental age groups (pregnancy to old age). The appendix also lists the professional services that are suggested for those same ten groups.

A final word about this guide. It is a mistake to think of it as a static document. Aircraft have flight plans which they follow if they can. But air traffic or weather may change so that completion of the plan as originally filed may be impossible. There is constant communication between flight controllers and the flight crew about position, progress, speed. And it works. The situation with personal health planning is entirely analogous. The original guide is just that—a guide. As the flight crew, you need to be in repetitive contact with your flight controllers (yourself, support people, your doctor, and other health providers) to assess progress, desirability of continuing through the same planned sequences to your destination. A guide is a flexible, changeable aid, not an inscribed stone tablet. The important thing is that you show progress. During some months or even years, it may be slow, but as long as you progress, you grow and become increasingly ready to do more to realize your potential.

Your Personal Health Guide will become part of your Self-Health Record, which is the subject of the next chapter. The Problem Lists, Strength Lists, Goals, Priorities, and Plans of the Guide will be the heart and guiding center for your Self-Health Record. What you decide to incorporate into the Progress section of the SHR will be directly determined by the priorities you elect in your plan. As you change priorities, add new problems, or resolve old ones, your plan will change correspondingly.

HEALTH FUELS ITSELF AND A GUIDE HELPS YOU BE HEALTHY

One of medicine's best kept secrets is that health begets more health. As people do things to promote and increase their own health, they have fewer illnesses and their effectiveness, efficiency, and joy in life increase. The following quote from Bloomfield and Kory emphasizes this idea:

On the basis of extensive research conducted over the last ten years on several thousand exceptionally healthy and long-lived individuals, we and a growing number of medical professionals believe that the health of the so-called healthy (in the sense of having a clean bill of health) individuals can be vastly improved. It appears that only a small fraction of the population currently enjoys anywhere near its full capacity for health. *Furthermore, this failure of people to make use of this capacity seems to be the single most important cause of much of today's illness.* To put it plainly, research is showing that by not achieving your full, natural measure of vigor and vitality, you invite not only unnecessary minor illness and unnecessarily rapid aging, but also heart attack, lung disease, and cancer, the most serious disease of our era.[3]

A carefully developed guide, used wisely, can help you move ever closer to your "full capacity for health." The next chapter will illustrate how the Personal Health Guide becomes an essential part of your Self-Health Record.

RESOURCES CHAPTER 3

Breslow and Somers. *The Lifetime Health-Monitoring Program* (see Appendix A). Provides health goals and recommended professional services for the major developmental age groups from pregnancy/perinatal to old age. Specific procedures are not included but criteria for selecting them are.

L.J. Weed, M.D. *Your Health Care and How to Manage It* (Essex Junction, VT: Essex Publishing Co.,1978) A detailed discussion of one approach to managing your health utilizing a self-kept record as the core activity.

3. Harold H. Bloomfield, and Robert B. Kory. *The Holistic Way to Health and Happiness: A New Approach to Complete Lifetime Wellness.* (New York: Simon and Schuster, 1978).

4

The Self-Health Record: Keeping Track

WALT sprang to his feet and moved quickly toward the vacant carpeted floor at the center of the group. "It's time to show you this," he said, unfurling an eight-foot roll of paper. "This is my blood pressure record over the last five years. Several years ago it looked like I might have a problem with high blood pressure. So I started to keep track of it myself." We saw two sawtooth lines running across the entire scroll. Within the first foot they gradually declined and then leveled off within normal range. "I've taken readings at times when I felt stressed and before and after exercise. I made a note of those things along the bottom here." Sure enough, he had made brief notations about weight, life events, diet, and exercise. "That way I discovered what I could do without medicine to keep my blood pressure normal."

With that dramatic, unrehearsed, surprise display of a self-initiated, self-designed, and clearly effective record, my first self-care group never questioned that maintaining a useful record of health practices and medical problems is one of the single most important things people can do to promote their health.

A main goal of health competence is to have you become more attentive to your health — to *pay attention*, to invest your life with attention. Building and maintaining a health record creates immediate, tangible involvement with your health. It's like keeping financial records. We have checking accounts, savings accounts, credit accounts, and mortgage accounts, and although not everyone is meticulous, most of us do maintain some kind of financial records. In general, the better our records are, the healthier our finances are. Even if we don't keep such records, the companies and institutions we are dealing with do. Our banks, mortgagors, and creditors all send us monthly statements. We wouldn't do business with them if they didn't.

With medical records, the general situation is much different. Every doctor and hospital with whom you have been a customer keeps a record (their quality varies tremendously) about you and your visits. Yet, usually *you* don't know what is in that record. If you are told, you are unlikely to remember clearly! If you're an average person, you haven't even asked for a copy of the "findings." Even when you moved and changed doctors you probably didn't ask for your records. Alas, people are far more conditioned to take care of their wealth (or lack of) than their health (or lack of).

THE BENEFITS OF A SELF-HEALTH RECORD

A Self-Health Record helps you be more attentive by reflecting (like video replay) in words and graphs what is going on. A good record makes problems clear, indicates change, and helps you choose the best options.

Your Self-Health Record permits you to own your data, to see it when you want to, to show it to others as you choose, including professionals. When

people do ask for facts or the reasons for decisions, these are usually given verbally and, consequently, often forgotten. Seldom are you apprised of the physician's thinking about your problem. In your own record, this can be done. This helps to strengthen self-responsibility.

The Self-Health Record helps initiate or improve communication with physicians or other health workers. Interactions can become more focused and fruitful. Also, a self-health record demystifies much of medicine, thereby lessening intimidation of many consumers. Everyone has encountered terms and procedures they never fully understood (see Figure 4-1, "The Doctor-Patient Communication Gap"). People let them slide by. If *you* are keeping a Record, you will be more stimulated to ask the doctor to explain matters in terms that are clear to you.

The Record can facilitate health maintenance and well-being. It shows areas in which you *could* be healthier, those where you *choose* to be healthier, and how you are progressing. It can include exercise records, dietary changes, assessments of life stress, and much more. Also, it will help you identify more clearly some of your barriers to health, some of the "old tapes" that impede you. It can help make you healthful!

The Record provides continuity to your story. Your life is a continuing story. If you don't consider the past plot, what

FIGURE 4-1   The Doctor-Patient Communication Gap.

The doctor says:	The patient thinks:	But really . . .
tumor	cancer	A mass or swelling not ordinarily found. It may be cancer, or it may be a non-cancerous growth, abcess, or swelling from trauma.
angina pectoris	heart attack	A chest pain of cardiac origin. It is serious, but not the same as having a heart attack.
cholecystectomy	huh?!	A gall bladder operation.

unfolds today may surprise you or make no sense at all. But if you pay attention, take notes, and think about how events connect, the story will make sense, and you may even be able to predict what is yet to occur. Unfortunately, for the vast majority of us, the whole story is not kept — not in one place, anyway.

Take Matthew, aged 25. His only operation was in New York City at age 4-1/2 months for a double hernia. Until age 10 he went to a private GP and belonged to a dental-care program. When he moved to a new town, his family switched to a health insurance/maintenance plan and a private dentist. Matthew attended three public schools in the new town before going to college. There, he regularly used the health service; on one occasion he was hospitalized overnight. After college he worked near Philadelphia, going to two different GP's when necessary. Since moving to Chicago he has seen a doctor and a dentist once each. In this brief history, 15 places are identified that have, or had, fragments of this young man's medical story. *The only complete version is in his own record.* Matthew's story is not unusual. Do you have a composite of your health and medical story?

Finally, *a Self-Health Record can save you time, money, and unnecessary risks.*

These benefits result from preventing duplication of tests and examinations and from reducing the number and duration of costly hospitalizations. Unnecessary duplication of x-rays is particularly important because of the well-documented risks of radiation. A record of allergies or troublesome side effects to your medications can prevent recurrences, saving time, money, and possibly your life! These benefits all multiply in this age of great geographic mobility. Over the years, the Record almost invariably supports Ben Franklin's maxim, "An ounce of prevention is worth a pound of cure."

Keeping a Self-Health Record is itself a wellness activity. The Record *may* lead you to exercise, to reduce your weight, or to cut down on smoking, alcohol, or coffee. If it doesn't, it is not a failure. The mere presence of a well-kept Record in your life — even in a life that essentially remains unchanged — can improve your health potential dramatically.

BUILDING A SELF-HEALTH RECORD (SHR)

The following diagram illustrates how the SHR is developed. For maximum effectiveness, your Self-Health Record will incorporate both your Self-Appraisal (Chapter 2) and your Personal Health

FIGURE 4–2   Diagram of the Self-Health Record.

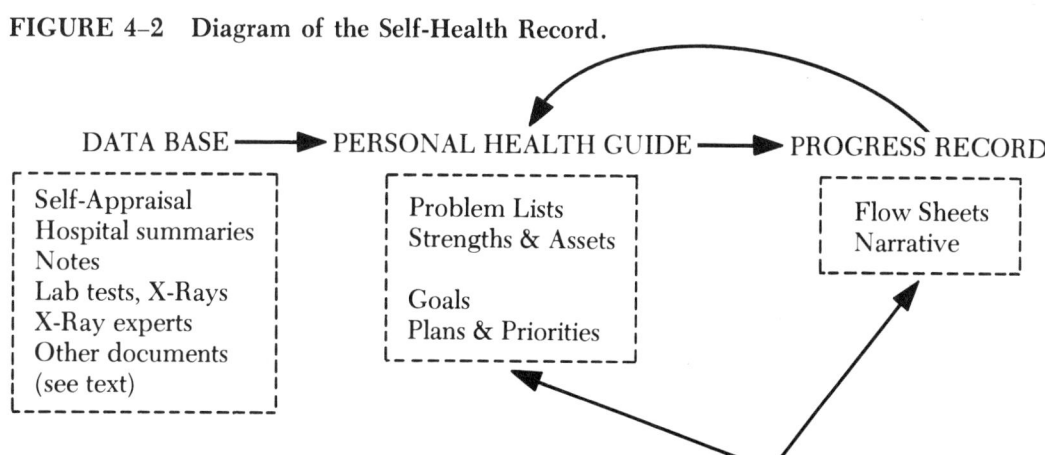

Guide, PHG, (Chapter 3). The appraisal becomes part of the data base. The PHG will become the guiding document for choosing and sequencing your health activities, and the record you keep of your progress. The record is a chronicle of what you actually do (and don't do) about your health and well-being. What you do and don't do, sensibly, will reflect your PHG.

A Self-Health Record can be kept in any organized system — in files, folders, or a loose-leaf notebook with dividers (I prefer the latter). Divide the Record into four sections labeled Data Base, Personal Health Guide, Progress, and Resources. Later you may wish to subdivide sections or create new ones. Their exact character is up to you. But these four sections give the best foundations without complications or confusion.

DATA BASE

The *Data Base* should contain any or all of the following as they can be acquired. The first items are all part of your completed self-appraisal if you have done it:

- A medical history of your illnesses, significant injuries, and important symptoms, including their management and treatment, and names of hospitals, doctors, and other health workers involved.
- A health hazard appraisal and wellness inventory; the health hazard appraisal identifies your "hidden" health problems and is Part III of your Self-Appraisal. The wellness inventory identifies your health habits and lifestyle practices, and is Part IV of your Self-Appraisal in Chapter 2.
- The family history answers basic health questions about parents, siblings, and other close relatives. This is in Part III of your Self-Appraisal.
- Major medical records covering hos-

pitalizations, important emergency room visits, and extended periods of care by one physician in his or her office. Summaries, if available, may provide all the information you need. If you are curious or the details are important, try to get the whole record.
- Lab results, X-ray reports, electrocardiograms, consultation reports.

To repeat, the Medical History, the Wellness Inventory, the Health Hazard Appraisal and the Family History are part of your Self-Appraisal. A physician may have completed all or some of them on you as well.

For hospitalizations or significant physician contacts in the past, requisition the records (or summaries) of those events. People are amazed to learn they can do this. At my urging a student successfully requisitioned her record from a local hospital. She was excited like a child with a new treasured toy — and considerably less mystified by what had happened during hospitalizations some years before! Summaries may provide all of the information you need, but if you are very curious or details are important, try to obtain the entire record. This is not easy in some states, and in a few it is not possible.

If a doctor or hospital initially declines to provide the information, don't give up or get angry immediately. Many institutions still have archaic rules concerning records disclosure. Write a cordial but firm letter to the doctor or the hospital administrator briefly explaining that you wish to have the information for your personal Record. If resistance continues, remain firm and begin to cite legal rights, referring to state law.

Unfortunately, state laws vary dramatically and sometimes favor institutions. Old-fashioned persistence is often more effective than falling back on the law. However, *Getting Yours: A Con-*

sumer's Guide to Obtaining Your Medical Record can give you a lot of help with facts on laws and good general advice[1].

Don't be discouraged if you cannot obtain your Data Base all at once. And don't wait to complete your Data Base before starting the rest of your Record.

As you collect information, remember that you are interested in maintaining and increasing health as well as dealing with problems and disease. The Record is *not* meant as an aid to hypochondria. A significant portion (for some people, *most*) of your data should reflect the positive aspect of your total effort. (Your wellness inventory is an example.)

PERSONAL HEALTH GUIDE (PROBLEMS, STRENGTHS, GOALS AND PLANS)

The Problems, Strengths, Goals, and Plans which you have defined as part of your Personal Health Guide (Chapter 3) summarizes in a page or two your present health status, medical history, and future health intentions. They are the heart of your self-health record, its table of contents, and they become the point of reference for the Progress and Resources sections of your Record.

If you are building your Self-Health Record without first having completed your Personal Health Guide, you must, as a minimum, have a Problem List (developed in the same way as described in the Personal Health Guide Chapter). If you have completed your Personal Health Guide, then you may want to supplement the problem lists in it from other parts of the Data Base (like your old hospital records). Remember that a Problems list can be made on the basis of any amount of data, however small or large, and *a problem is anything you perceive to be a problem*. It may be a symptom (headache, knee pain, nervousness),

a doctor's diagnosis (gallstones, appendicitis), an abnormal exam finding (lump in breast), or a lab test finding (high cholesterol). Label problems in words you understand (e.g., "high blood pressure" instead of "hypertension").

Your Problems List in the PHG will also include those habits you may wish to change or those you know are less than healthy (your potential problems). Examples include smoking, excessive drinking, lack of exercise, not wearing seat belts. These are health maintenance problems. Such matters may not cause trouble now, but may eventually result in medical difficulties; you should be aware of them.

Don't be concerned or frustrated if your list seems long. Ten to 30 problems for a middle-aged adult is not unusual, though many of these problems will be minor or inactive. It helps give both you and any health providers with whom you share the list a total picture of you and your health status, and helps you choose wisely the problems to work with at the present time.

Most important, be honest! The primary reason for a Self-Health Record is to depict your true health status.

The Strengths and Assets lists in your PHG should reflect what you and others see as your personal strong points, as well as your advantages in life — using the financial analogy again, your assets. Typical examples are "savings: $3,600," "well-conditioned," and "strong support from wife." Too often people muddle through problems without mobilizing their strengths to help cope. Having that list of positive attributes in front of you makes strengths harder to forget.

Your PHG will indicate which problems you wish to work on for the next few months. Do any problems absolutely override all others? Cancer is an extreme example. Insulin-dependent diabetes is another problem that must be dealt with

---

1. See Resources for this chapter.

regularly. If you have such an insistent problem, it will surely be your top priority.

PROGRESS RECORD

So far, you have focused on your problems and strengths in general, set priorities, and organized your thinking on individual problems. It is time to address them in the most systematic, reasonable, and effective manner possible to reach your goals. The Progress section will help you do that.

The plans portion of your PHG serves as the springboard for the Progress section of the Self-Health Record. Your working plans (and their implied priorities) provide the mechanism for choosing those problems both present and potential which you will work on. If you work on them they need a progress record.

All Progress Notes (don't forget those health maintenance/wellness "potential" problems) should be kept in an appropriately labeled subdivider or folder filed by problem (e.g., "sleeplessness" or "abdominal pain"). They may take two forms: 1) an outline or narrative, or 2) a flow sheet — a table or graph that records certain important data over time.

The outline or narrative note is illustrated in Figure 4-3. As a rule, each narrative progress note reflects in its data section what happened as a result of the plan in the previous note. The first progress note records what has happened since the plan in the PHG. Current thinking and plans are also given if these have changed. The data recorded in a Progress Note is of two types:

1. What you are feeling; how your symptoms have changed.
2. Findings on the physical examination, laboratory data, X-ray reports, biopsies, etc., and any data you have obtained yourself, such as weight, blood pressure, temperature.

In the example, all of the data is on the first type. It should be re-emphasized that the *thinking* (both your own and the physician's or other health worker's) about a problem should include any unanswered questions that may be in your mind.

In the *plan* of the progress note, you must consider further steps to diagnose the condition, if necessary, as well as treatment and educational needs. It is helpful to number them. "Figuring out" steps and treatment steps need not be separated since some plans are both anyway. For instance, to deal with sleeplessness, a person may decide to stop drinking coffee; this may turn out to be both a diagnostic step and a therapeutic one!

All Progress Notes do not necessarily contain data, thinking, and plans. If there is no new data, that line can be omitted or you may simply write, "Data: none."

Flow sheets and graphic progress notes are best used with problems where repeated observations are made over a short period of time (e.g., diabetes, hypertension, overweight, anxiety). With some imagination, the progress of most problems can be recorded in this simplified manner. Flow sheets provide a tangible, visual image of involvement, which appeals to most people.

Flow sheets have several advantages. First, one sheet can record progress over a long period. You may be able to keep a year's progress data on one flow sheet, as opposed to many narrative sheets. Second, numerical data from studies is best handled in this way. Certain key items from the historical and physical data can also be recorded. You can see changes (or no changes) along one line; there is no

FIGURE 4–3   Progress Notes of Self-Health Record.

Progress Notes (narrative)

Problem: Toothache, jaw pain

(Started this sheet on 15th)

Data	Assessment	Plan
13 May 81 – Slight toothache in right upper molar		Taking aspirin
14 May 81 – toothache worse, sometimes pain in nearby teeth	Infected tooth?	Continuing aspirin, using Ambesol
15 May 81 – pain increasing: an intermittant, pulsing pain; aching beginning to appear in cheek and jaw joint. Aspirin, Ambesol help little	Joint problem?	Trying Tylenol (extra-strength); continuing Ambesol trying to relax
16 May 81 – dramatic increase in pain, impossible to concentrate on work. Ambesol no longer works. – Later: Empirin makes pain worse	This isn't psychosomatic. things are doing well, other than this	Trying Empirin w/ codeine – back to Tylenol
17 May 81 – tooth pain has spread throughout right side, upper and lower; jaw joint severe; sleeping very difficult (must sleep on left side w/ head raised); right jaw visibly swollen	Could it be a nerve problem? Seems more mouth oriented still, but may not be at this point	Continuing Tylenol. Appt. w/dentist (18). If he doesn't find anything, may then try M.D.

need to flip from page to page (see Figure 4-4). Finally, once the flow sheet is established, recording observations requires less time.

At the risk of being repetitive, *don't forget your health maintenance problems.* Choose at least one to deal with over the next six months, and design a flow sheet that will help you work on the problem.

As you chart and describe your progress, keep your mind open. Don't condemn or judge data too quickly. Consider whether the data proves 1) that the plans outlined in your PHG were reasonable, 2) that you are indeed progressing, and

FIGURE 4-4   Flow Sheet for Self-Health Record.
Flow Sheet

Date/Time	B.P.*	Pulse	WT	Meds/Dose	Exercise	Other Comments	Symptoms	Thinking	Plans
7/16–30/78	160/110 170/110 165/105	80 82 85	178	none	none	uses lots of salt	irritable, tense headache	evaluation complete needs treatment	treat with hygroton (H), ismelin later if necessary; lose weight, exercise
8/7/78	170/100	82	179	H25/d	walk 2m/day		same	start treatment	see in 1 month; call if have questions
9/5/78	150/95	78	176	H25/d	walk 3m/day	using less salt	some headaches, less tense	some good change in B.P.	same except increase vigor of exercise. See in 1 month.
10/8/78	140/90	78	174	H25/d	walk 3m/day runs 2m-3x week		headaches improved	progressing well	pursue weight loss, move vigorously; learn 1500 cal diet
11/6/78	130/55	75	168	H25/d	same	enjoys exercise sticking to diet	feeling "good"	coming along well, don't change anything now	no change in plan

Name – JOHN JONES   Height – 5'8"   Problem: High Blood Pressure

+ H = hygroton
*BP = blood pressure taken in right arm sitting down

3) that you have been addressing the correct problem.

At intervals, and no later than at the end of the time span set in your initial goal, sit down with the PHG and the Progress Notes and evaluate your situation fully. Record your revised plan (or the same plan if the initial one is working).

When a problem is resolved, reaches a less pressing stage, or begins to be managed as part of your natural daily routine, return to your Problems List. Pick the next most pressing or important problem(s) and begin the process again.

The Progress section reflects the nature of the whole record and your whole life. It is ongoing. At first this may be disconcerting. Unlike high school or college, it doesn't end, and you don't graduate. After a while, this becomes a plus of the Self-Health Record for many people. It doesn't contain rigid goals, *per se*.

RESOURCES

The last section of the Self-Health Record, the *Resources*, can be highly individualized both in content and format. In general, it includes all helpful information you find concerning your active problems. It may contain newspaper or magazine articles, pamphlets, booklets, and reference lists to books or other bulky materials on your bookshelf or in a library. Or it may contain the phone numbers to various health-care personnel or hotlines. Include resources relating to health maintenance and well-being.

OBTAINING YOUR MEDICAL RECORDS

It is often important to requisition copies or summaries of your medical records from physician(s) or hospital(s). These records can become an important part of your data base. You can also find out what has been said about you and your

illness and be better prepared to protect your privacy.

The Federal Privacy Act assures access to records from a federal hospital (public health service, Veterans Administration, or military). Where other hospitals are concerned, your legal rights will vary considerably. In many states, there is no legislation providing access to records, which doesn't necessarily mean that you can't get them. (See Appendix B). In states where access is legally granted, it may be limited in a number of ways.

However unfavorable the legal situation may be in the state concerned, a given hospital or physician may be very willing to provide copies. Existing laws are more often permissive than restrictive. Reluctance to surrender records is more likely to relate to "prevailing practice standards" than clear legal constraints. Therefore, *don't be discouraged* from attempting to get records because the state has restrictive legislation or none at all.

Always proceed with the confidence that the information in that record *is yours* — it is from and about you. Whether it is interview data, answers to questionnaires, physical exam data, laboratory work, or X-rays, *it is all your data*. If the health provider is unwilling to surrender your own information, he will with few exceptions have difficulty in defending the position legally, no matter what state laws say.

SUMMARY OF LEGAL SITUATIONS IN VARIOUS STATES

Appendix B summarizes the current legal status in the individual states. This information is taken from *Medical Records: Getting Yours* a publication of the Health Research Group, Washington, D.C. This guide is recommended to those who wish more detail than is provided in this book (see Resources).

APPROACH TO GETTING YOUR RECORDS

The following approach for obtaining your records is largely modified from *Medical Records: Getting Yours.* It works and has been successfully employed by many people.

1. *Before doing anything, know your rights* (Appendix B) and the usual community practice. Learn about the latter by asking friends, calling the medical record librarian or "patient advocate" at the hospital, or phoning the county medical society. You may find there is little or no information available on either legal rights or usual practice.

2. *Know what part of the record you want.* If you have a large record, you may only want a summary or a specific section (such as the history, physical exam, lab or X-ray reports) rather than the entire file. If possible, arrange to inspect the record and choose the parts you need. This will also save money, since most hospitals and physicians charge to copy records. If the record is not very large, it is best to ask for the entire record.

3. *Contact the doctor or hospital involved.* Have a summary of your legal rights (if any) and local practice in front of you. Say clearly what you want and ask what steps are necessary for you to take. Make a written request, if that is necessary. You may be asked to sign a release form. Although usually straightforward, read it carefully. If you have *any* doubts about signing, such as your right to prosecute the health provider after signing, contact a lawyer.

4. *Be patient, persevere.* If your inquiry meets with resistance or "passing the buck," pursue whatever steps are suggested. If you are told flatly you cannot obtain your records, submit a written request with the following information:

Your name, date of birth.
Dates you were hospitalized or under the care of the physician.
A statement like this: "I would like to have a copy of my entire medical record for my hospitalization, 1/17/-80–1/23/80," or "I want a copy of all of Dr. Smith's office notes from the period of March 1976 to December 1980."

State that you are willing to pay reasonable copying costs and to sign a request form if necessary.
Enclose a list of your legal rights, if you know what they are.

5. *If your written request is denied or not answered, seek assistance.* If there is no hurry, wait a month before taking further action. If you need the records immediately to facilitate care of a current problem by another doctor or hospital, enlist their aid immediately. Providers seldom refuse transfer of records to other providers. If there is still difficulty try patients' rights groups. Women's groups, minority organizations, or groups for the elderly (such as the Grey Panthers) may provide good help. If necessary, have a lawyer make the request on your behalf if you think the additional cost is worthwhile. A lawyer can be helpful if the avenues listed above have failed. Threatened lawsuits often work. Actual lawsuits are likely to be fruitful only if the right to access is legalized in state law. Things are changing. It is already more commonplace for people to ask for their records. The right to access will become legally validated in more and more states, and will soon, I believe, prevail generally. The fundamental rightness of your requests will be in-

creasingly recognized, no matter what the legal status in your state now.

HOW TO EXAMINE YOUR RECORD ONCE YOU HAVE IT

Naturally, each person will have different kinds of information he or she would like to find in the record. Reports of specific lab tests and X-rays are a common example. Once you have such a record, however, you may help yourself (and your future health) a lot if you examine it carefully to answer the following questions:

1. When a diagnosis (name, label, problem name) is made, what was the basis (evidence) on which it was made?
2. For the various lab tests and X-rays, medications, and surgical procedures that were used, is it clear why they were done? Is the reasoning clear from the information in the record? (Usually it is not.) Do you have any reason to believe (or not believe) that alternatives were considered that might have been more effective, less expensive, or less dangerous?
3. Did the treatments used (medication, surgery, other things like physical therapy) help or not help to resolve the problem?
4. Is there any evidence of allergic reactions or other bad reactions to any medicine that you were not informed about at the time (or since)?

As you examine the record with these questions in mind, note whatever is unclear, and write down any questions you may have. Use books, your pharmacist, any patient advocate, knowledgeable friends, your physician, and other health professionals in trying to resolve any confusion and to answer your questions.

Like any new program or system, creating a Self-Health Record involves some initial time and nominal expense. Both with patience and perseverance, the Record will soon reward you. And you need no special skills or background to do it.

Every Record will have its own variations, its own personality. What has been presented here is a basic framework from which you can create what works most effectively for you. People who are trying to lose weight often find that an eating record is very useful. An exercise log is also popular, particularly with runners. And some people find that keeping an intensive journal or diary is beneficial; it can be an important adjunct to emotional/spiritual wellness; and a Self-Health Record addresses far more than just physical health. It can enrich your whole life.

Remember that your health record can be a creative tool. The structure outlined here will keep it orderly as your record expands. If you wish, supplement and enrich that structure with any ideas that will truly make it your own.

RESOURCES CHAPTER 4

M. Sarath, M. Auerback, and T. Bogue. *Medical Records: Getting Yours: A Consumer's Guide to Obtaining Your Medical Record.* An excellent publication of the Health Research Group, Dept. MR, 200 P. St., N.W., Washington, D.C. 20036.

P. Ways and J.W. Jones. *The Problem Oriented Medical Record: A Self-Instructional Unit.* Health Sciences Consortium, 200 Easttowne Drive, Chapel Hill, N.C. 27514. (919) 942-8731.

Weed. *Your Health and How to Manage It.* (see previous chapter).

5

Gathering and Describing Health Information

GATHERING information is basic to most complex activities. Attaining and maintaining good health and well-being is no exception to this statement. With respect to health, the most basic information comes from our own minds, spirits, and bodies. Three kinds of skills are essential to gathering and using that data: self-awareness, examination, and description. Recognizing and clearly perceiving what is happening in your mind, body, and spirit are the essence of *self-awareness* skills. Evaluating and estimating the activities and state of body parts by looking, feeling, and using certain simple instruments are the *examination skills*. The skill of clearly *describing* your perceptions and the results of your examinations is equally important. If you can't accurately describe an awareness or the findings on examination, part of their value is lost. These three skills, self-awareness, examination, and describing, are interdependent and overlapping. Proficiency in any one enhances the others. A fourth skill, *focused knowledge search*, comes into play after you have formulated some initial impressions about what is going on. The relationship of these four skills of information gathering is shown in Figure 5-1.

SELF-AWARENESS SKILLS

Self-awareness or "tuning-in" is the ability to recognize and interpret important mind-body messages. Not everyone finds this an easy task, and it is one that requires practice, inventiveness, and attentiveness. The perception of bodily

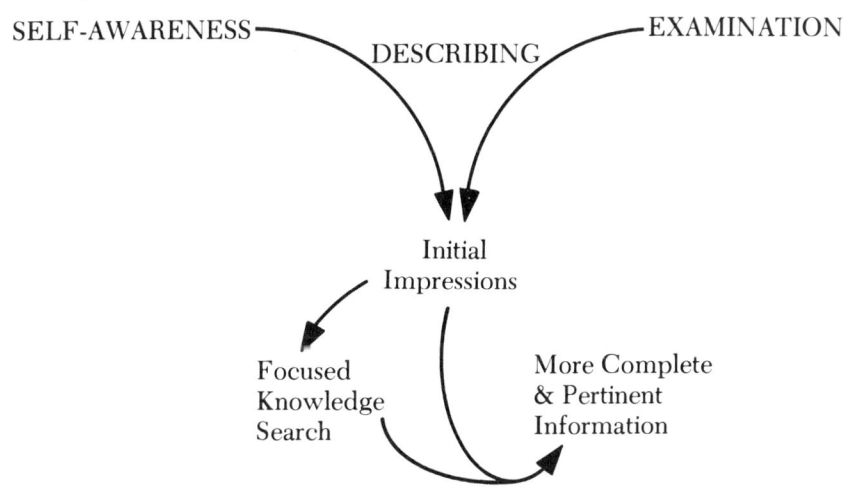

FIGURE 5–1   The Relationship of the Four Skills of Information Gathering.

sensations, thoughts, and feelings is the essential first step. Pain, achiness, fatigue, tightness in the shoulders, nausea, and tension may all be manifestations of physical and emotional discord.

Assessment of energy reserves through self-awareness is also particularly important. Starting a new activity or increasing the intensity of an old one requires good energy supplies. Fatigue, listlessness, lack of humor, and outright depression may all be indicators of low energy.

"Tuning in" can be facilitated by several strategies. One is a journal. Getting closer to a troubling experience by writing about it often awakens feelings or emotions that were previously unconscious. Another strategy is to think about yourself and your experiences during aerobic exercise (running, swimming) or after meditating or yoga. Thinking is much clearer and new ideas are more freely generated during exercise and after meditation. This requires enough conditioning or meditative skills to sustain the activity for 20–30 minutes.

For many people, however, talking with a friend or a confidant is the best tool for increasing awareness. It also helps directly in learning to describe things. Many people hardly ever express strong emotions and feelings to anyone. They don't *reflect on* their experiences, which is different than simply *reflecting* the experience.

Self-awareness in the spiritual realm is stimulated and enhanced by meditation or prayer, or some other means of communion with yourself and whatever spiritual power you acknowledge. I think of these activities as talking to a spiritual friend or to a friendly and supportive spirit.

BASIC EXAMINING SKILLS

The examination skills are just that. They involve looking, hearing, and feeling with your hands and making measurements with simple instruments—the thermometer, the bathroom scale, the blood pressure apparatus (sphygmomanometer). Some looking involves instruments—the flashlight, tongue blade, stethoscope, and the otoscope (for looking into the ears). People in self-care groups become competent with these procedures. They love this part of the class; somehow these skills represent activities which had been previously relegated to the exclusive realm of the physician/magician.

Some of the basic examination skills described below are difficult to carry out on yourself. For example, unless you are a remarkable contortionist, examining your own ear is essentially impossible. Compared to the throat and skin, which are easy to examine for most of us, the self-exam of the abdomen is also difficult, but a lot can be learned even if the exam cannot be done exactly as described. However, Personal Health Competence involves caring for others as well as yourself. So learning to examine ears or abdomens can be helpful in that way.

One word of caution. Many people (including, alas, medical students and doctors) become so fascinated with instruments that they neglect their unaided powers of observation. It is amazing how much can be observed with the unaided eye and hands. Work hard on it and you will be pleased at the results. I have seen medical students fail to detect a significant abdominal mass or note weakness of one arm, because they were so preoccupied with using their badges of office, the eyescope and the heartscope.

One of the hardest things is learning what is "normal" and what is not. This requires examining a number of people. If you think you have found something unusual on yourself or another person, it is good practice to check it on someone else who is well. Your doctor or her nurse may help, and good books on physical examination are also important (see resources). Examining normal people is the best way to learn what is usual and what is not.

Basic Examining Skills

How to Take Temperature

Temperature can be taken with the thermometer in the mouth under the tongue, in the armpit (axillary), and in the anus (rectal). The rectal route is most accurate for small children and infants but must be done carefully to avoid breakage of

the thermometer with sudden movements (see Figure 5-2). Some children will not tolerate a rectal thermometer. The armpit method is good but tends not to be as accurate as the others. It is best for children who will cooperate well and who are intolerant of the oral or rectal route.

Clean the thermometer well before and after use. Don't take temperature within half an hour of eating, drinking, or smoking. Keep the thermometer in place three minutes for oral and rectal readings, and five for axillary. Make sure the thermometer reads below 97° when you begin. If it does not, lower the reading by placing it under cold water for sufficient time or by shaking it down with a wrist snapping motion. Read the thermometer in a good light. Grasp the end of the thermometer opposite the mer-

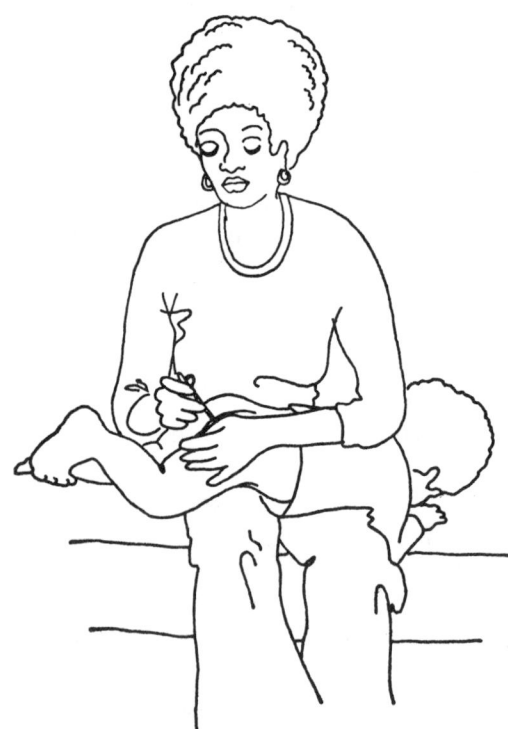

FIGURE 5–2   Taking a Rectal Temperature.

Grateful acknowledgement is made to Healthwise, Inc., of Boise, Idaho, for permission to reproduce six drawings (Figures 5-2 through 5-7) from the *Healthwise Handbook, The Practical Guide to Family-Based Care,* 4th Edition, Healthwise, Inc., Boise, Idaho, 1983.

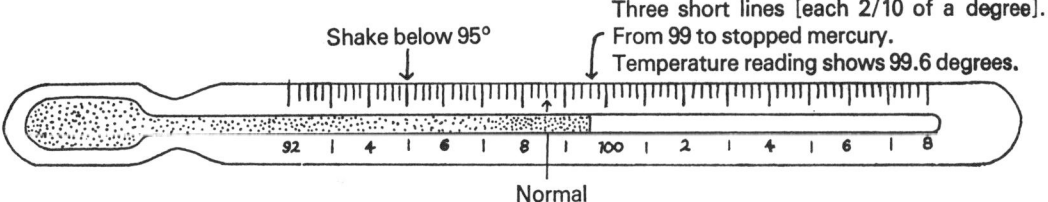

FIGURE 5-3   Reading a Thermometer.

cury bulb between thumb and forefinger and rotate it slowly until you see the ribbon of mercury — it may be silver or red (see Figure 5-3). Wherever the ribbon stops is the temperature reading. Write down the reading, the date and time, and the method used to take the temperature (oral, rectal, axillary).

With the oral method, make sure the thermometer is under the tongue and the mouth closed. When doing the axillary method hold the upper arm in tightly against the thermometer. The rectal thermometer should be inserted through the anus but no further (usually about two thirds of the thermometer is still visible when the cheeks of the buttock are held aside). It should be held lightly with the thumb and forefinger the entire time that it is in place. It may be most convenient to hold children in your lap, face down, while taking their rectal temperature.

Measuring the Pulse Rate

Except in an emergency or when it is being used to measure the heart rate during exercise, the pulse is taken after the subject has been sitting or lying quietly for a minute or two. A pulse can be taken wherever an artery comes close to the skin surface. Usually it is taken at the wrist, but often it's easier to feel in the neck.

To take the pulse at the wrist, place two fingers (never your thumb) against the wrist as shown in Figure 5-4. Bending the wrist slightly may make it easier to feel the pulsations. Count the beats for 30 seconds then multiply the results by two. The pulse is recorded in beats per

minute. As you count the pulse, keep your fingers on the artery and feel for regularity. Does the pulse speed up or slow down or skip beats? In many normal people, the pulse will be faster as they breathe in and slower as they breathe out. Record the rate and regularity.

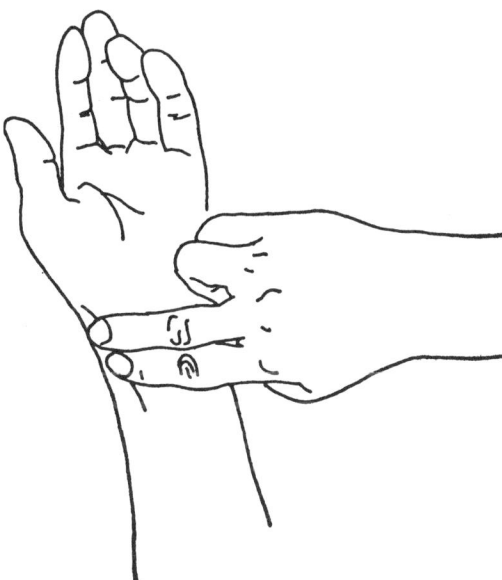

FIGURE 5-4   Taking a Pulse Rate.

If it is hard to feel a throbbing at the wrist, place two fingers at the side of the voice box and slide them back into the groove between the muscles and the voice box while turning the head slightly to the same side. Then you should feel the carotid pulse. Go ahead and experiment — you do not have to press very hard if your fingers are in the correct place. (Sometimes in an emergency you cannot determine the pulse at the wrist or the neck; if so, put your ear or a stethoscope to the person's chest and count the beats as you hear them.)

The normal heart rate is 60–80 in the resting adult (even slower rates are found in many well-trained athletes), 70–110 in 6–10 year olds, and 70–150 in babies.

Taking Blood Pressure

For routine checks and periodic monitoring, it is essential to take the blood pressure in the same position and the same arm each time. The best position for the subject is sitting in a chair with the arm across the corner of table. This allows the arm to relax and assures the same vertical relationship between the subject's heart and the point at which the blood pressure is measured each time it is taken. The apparatus used for taking blood pressure is shown in Figure 5-5.

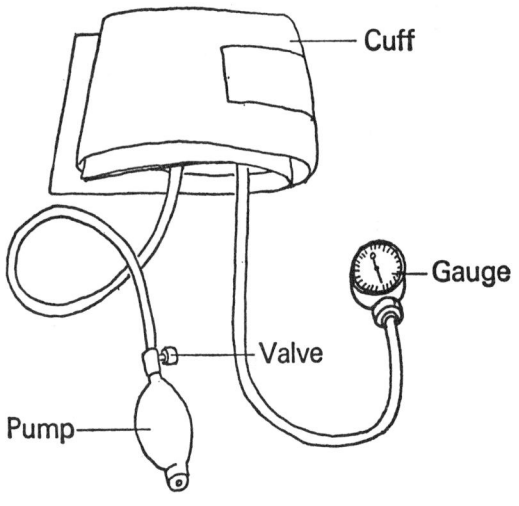

FIGURE 5–5   Blood Pressure Cuff.

The correct size cuff should be used: a children's cuff for small arms, a standard cuff for most people, and a large cuff for large arms. Cuffs vary in the way they are held in place around the arm. Most now have a velcro fastening. The cuff should fit snugly around the upper arm with the lower margin of the cuff one inch above the fold of skin inside the elbow. The bell or diaphragm (the latter works best) of the stethoscope is placed over the center of the fold or a little toward the outside. Experiment until you find the place where the sounds are clearest. The first time you take anyone's blood pressure (including your own), pump the cuff up until the dial reads 160 or more (with children 140). If you then hear pulse sounds through the stethoscope continue pumping until the sounds disappear. Then let the air slowly out while listening for the pulse sounds. The needle will usually begin to bounce before you can hear the sounds. The reading on the dial which corresponds to the first pulse sound you hear is the upper blood pressure (systolic) reading. Continue to let the air out slowly until the sounds disappear. That is the lower or diastolic reading. Let the cuff deflate completely and repeat the procedure. However, the second time only pump up the cuff until the dial reads 20 points higher than the systolic reading you got the first time. Take your readings again. If the second readings are more than 4–5 points different from the first set (either systolic or diastolic), repeat the readings a third (and if necessary) a fourth time. It is best if you can get a nurse or doctor to show you how to do blood pressures the first time and check out the readings you obtain with those they get. Instructions are usually included with the blood pressure apparatus and should be followed as well.

Taking your own blood pressure is usually not too difficult. Equipment is sold with the diaphragm of the stethoscope sewn right into the blood pressure cuff. Even if you don't have that kind of equipment, it is possible to tuck the diaphragm under the cuff so it will be held there as the cuff is inflated. Pump up the cuff with your free hand. Get someone to help you the first few times.

A person's blood pressure reading

should be the average of those taken at various times of the day under various conditions. In an adult, normal pressure is below 140 systolic and 90 diastolic. However, normal pressures in an adult can go as low as 90/50. Continued readings of more than 90 diastolic and/or 140 systolic should be discussed with your doctor and checked by someone else who has experience.

Measuring Respiratory Rate

It is best to measure respiration after you (or your subject) have been resting for a full minute. Do it by watching the rise and fall of the chest. Try to "breathe normally." Some people will breathe faster when they know you are measuring their respiratory rate. The normal respiratory rate in adults is from 8 to 20 per minute, and the higher levels (above 16) are usually only present when the person is anxious, unless there is a significant problem of some kind which is elevating the respiratory rate. Up to 30 breaths per minute is normal for children and 40 is for babies. Fever can raise the rate of respiration. If a person is wheezing or has obvious difficulty breathing this can mean asthma, pneumonia, or heart disease.

Examining the Throat

Examining the throat and inside of the mouth can be very helpful if you or someone else has fever, sore throat, cough, runny nose, headache, or any of those symptoms in combination. You'll need a bright light and the handle of a spoon to depress the tongue. Using a mirror you may be able to see the back of your throat without depressing your tongue. If examining someone else, get them to try that first also. It sometimes helps with children to have them pant forcibly with their tongue out or down. Everybody's mouth and throat looks a little different, so as with other parts of the exam, it pays

to look at a lot of them until you get good at identifying the various structures shown in the diagram. The more you can get help from someone who is practiced, the faster you will learn. You are looking for unusual areas of redness in the posterior pharynx, uvula, soft palate, and tonsils (if present). (See Figure 5-6.) Also look for swelling or white or yellow pus in all of the same areas. In smokers the back of the throat (and often the whole mouth) can be more red than usual.

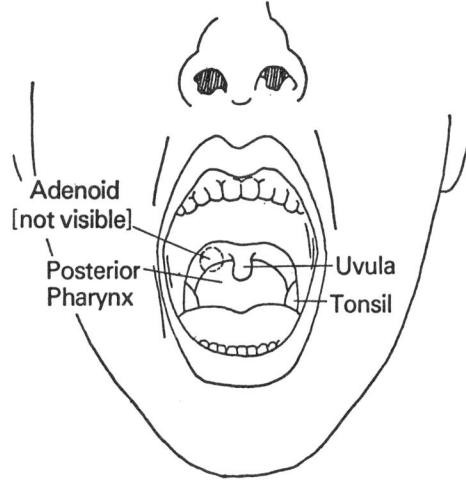

FIGURE 5-6 Mouth and Throat.

Examining the Ears

This is a particularly important exam when people have fever which is not obviously explained. Pull the ear gently to see if it causes pain. Look in the ear with a penlight, look for redness, pus, or wax. If you have an earscope (otoscope), do that exam while pulling up and backward on the earlobe. Find a diagram of the eardrum so that you can tell better what you are seeing. Exam of the eardrum and its interpretation is difficult. It is best to get help when you learn it and the first few times you do it. Hearing in the two ears can be compared by checking the distance from the ear at which a watch can be heard. Start with the watch against the ear and ask the person to tell you when the watch is no longer heard. Then move it slowly away from the ear until they say they can't hear it. Repeat once or twice to get a more accurate estimate. Then do it on the other ear. Some cases of ear damage or dysfunction where one side is more affected than the other can be detected in this way.

Examining the Skin

The important thing about examining the skin is to do all of it. It is the only organ that is entirely visible to the naked eye, since it is entirely on the outside of the body. To examine yourself, you may need another person or a mirror to help you see it all. As a routine matter you are looking for rashes, sores, and bumps. You need to examine the bottom of the feet, between the buttocks, in the groin, under the arms. Between fingers and toes, behind the ears, and the hair are other important areas to include. For maintaining health, the important thing is to notice any new skin changes that have occurred since the last time you did the examination. If there is a new sore or bump always feel for enlarged lymph nodes in the nearby area and in the armpits, front of the elbows, groin, back of the neck, and back of the knee, if any of those areas are near the new sore or bump.

It is important to write down your findings the first time you examine yourself or another person; you will never remember accurately.

Examining the Belly

The basic exam of the belly (abdomen) is in order to determine if there are any tender or hard places or to find out if the intestines are moving. To record what you find, imagine the abdomen to be divided into four parts by a vertical and horizontal line through the belly button.

These four areas are called the abdominal quadrants (right and left upper, right and left lower).

The person being examined should be undressed to the level of the groin. The exam should be done with the person on their back with knees bent and feet flat on the exam table so that tension on the front of the abdomen is at a minimum. Babies and young children normally have pot bellies. The exam with the hands is begun away from any part of the abdomen where the person is feeling pain or soreness. By the time the exam is completed, you should have made two complete circuits of the abdomen, going from one quadrant to another. (See Figure 5-7.) The first time around you press definitely but gently; the pressure should be about that of a grapefruit lying on your fingertips. The second time around you press in as deeply as possible. In painful areas it may not be possible to press in very far. If the person resists your

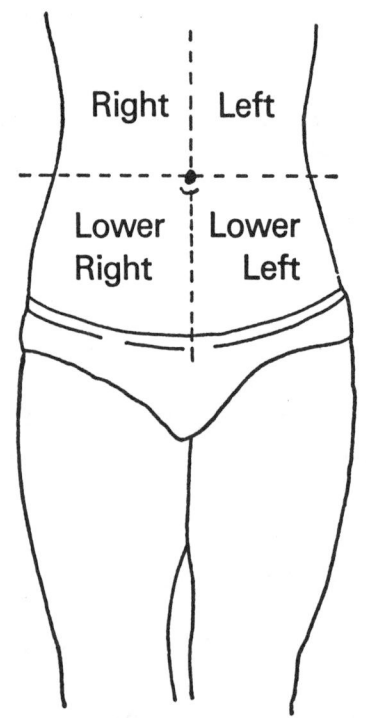

FIGURE 5-7   Abdominal Quadrants.

pressure by tightening the muscles of the abdomen, have him or her breath more deeply and relax. Record where there is tenderness, where it feels harder than in other places, and where there are lumps and bumps, if you feel any.

Listening can be done with a stethoscope or the naked ear. If you use the stethoscope just let it lie diaphragm down on the abdomen so you will not hear the sounds of your fingers rubbing against it. You are listening for gurgling sounds and little squeaks. The amount you hear will vary a lot. Normally everyone has sounds. If there are no sounds over two minutes time and the person has pain in the abdomen something serious may be happening.

FOCUSED KNOWLEDGE SEARCH

Beginners (of any age!) often wonder which problems to learn about first. Focused knowledge search means letting your study efforts be dictated by the situation rather than studying randomly. It also means using your self-awareness and examining skills first if appropriate. If you have a pain in your neck and run to look up pains in the neck, you may have an interesting time, but your efforts may be frustrating. If, by contrast, you take the time to appreciate that the pain is in the mid-left side, that you were painting the ceiling yesterday, that the muscles in the area of the pain feel hard and hurt more when you press on them, and that the pain is helped a little by aspirin but more by massaging the painful area, your reading session will be much more profitable. Chronic problems such as hypertension, arthritis, nervousness, or normal prolonged events like a pregnancy, or responsibilities for children or seniors, all provide good potential areas of focus.

This is not to say that reading medical and health books for curiosity and pleasure is not okay; it certainly is. But

don't depend on your memory about something you read last week, month, or year to help you with the current problem, unless it is repetitive or chronic and you are thoroughly knowledgeable about it. Knowledge for knowledge's sake is a fine thing. But what you learn by seeking and applying it directly to a problem today will definitely increase your health competence. It often takes just a few minutes.

DESCRIBING SKILLS

Describing skills are primarily facilitated and improved by talking with a confidant or keeping a journal. More specifically, your ability to describe what you experience will be improved by paying attention to its location (this is easy to picture for a symptom such as pain, but even with emotions it is often possible to identify a part of the body from which a sensation seems to come), how long it lasts, what seems to make it start, stop, get worse, or improve, its quality (sharp, dull, pleasant, unpleasant), intensity, and whether or not it is steady or seems to cycle from worse to better. This skill is enhanced by practicing your attentiveness to each of the items listed above. In Chapter 17 (The Beliefs and Skills of Health Partnership) the describing skills are explained in more detail as part of "telling your story." In general, people do not describe things accurately. Here is one good way to practice. Enlist the help of one or two friends. Together observe a person or event for just a few minutes and then, in just two minutes, each write a description of what occurred. Compare what each of you has written and notice differences. The next time have one person do the description verbally and then comment. By doing this three to four times a week for only a few weeks, alternating written and verbal descriptions, your description skills will improve greatly.

This review of the basic skills of information gathering and description is placed early in the book so that you can refer to it as you read other chapters. Probably in the course of the next few months you or someone close to you will have an illness or a health problem. Remember to use these skills to help work it out. As you apply them, their value will become rapidly apparent.

RESOURCES CHAPTER 5

1. Ryan and Travis. *Wellness Workbook* (see General Resources).

2. Roberts, Tinker, and Kemper. *Healthwise Handbook* (see General Resources). Particularly useful for examining skills.
3. Sehnert and Eisenberg. *How To Be Your Own Doctor (Sometimes)* (see General Resources). Also useful for the examination skills.
4. Werner. *Where There is No Doctor* (see General Resources). Chapter 3 is on examining a sick person.

Part ***III***

THE PATHWAY OF EMOTIONAL-SPIRITUAL HEALTH

EMOTIONAL-Spiritual health is at the core of health competence and of health. Although new books on various aspects of this subject appear constantly, their very number testifies that there is no one set of answers, no single right way of acquiring emotional-spiritual health. The views and suggestions which are made in these chapters have emerged from my own experience, reading, listening, and reflection on the behavior of others. As guidelines, they are working for me as well as for friends, colleagues, and clients.

Most of the precepts presented here are not my own. Many have been rediscovered for hundreds of years by various philosophers, religious figures, and psychotherapists. Although they may be expressed somewhat differently than you have experienced them before, they are mostly time-tested wisdom.

This pathway lays out a construct of emotional-spiritual health. I begin here, rather than with eating, moving, and habits, because the health of mind and spirit is fundamental. A person may have an injured or handicapped body, but if his mind is healthy and his spirit vibrant and strong, he will not only heal faster, he will feel well and strong as he does and will learn from that. On the other hand, if the spirit is weak or deranged, the emotions sickly, then no amount of body conditioning and healthy nutrition can bring true well-being. In fact, the person who is spiritless or crooked in spirit, who is emotionally confused, ambivalent, or terribly angry will probably not have the discipline and energy to achieve good physical conditioning or to maintain himself on a nutritious diet.

This part begins with a discussion of the mind-body connection and then formulates the guidelines for individual emotional-spiritual health and healthy relationships. The support of others is an integral part of health competence. Since

61

that idea is so difficult for some to accept and use effectively, and because such acceptance is an emotional-spiritual phenomenon, the last chapter in this part is "Advocacy and People Support Systems."

There is no chapter here (or elsewhere in this book) devoted specifically to stress and stress management. Stress is indeed an integral part of our lives. It is an essential source of energy for love and good works. When excessive or short-circuited in unhelpful ways it becomes dysfunctional, i.e., a source of *dis-ease* and an important factor in the causation and severity of many illnesses.

I believe the proper maintenance of emotional-spiritual health can minimize or eliminate dysfunctional stress. The principles outlined here in Part III as well as in Chapters 11–13 (covering body alignment, exercise, and sound nutrition) will do the job. In addition, Chapter 20 (Alternatives to Medicine and Surgery. Why Not?) has a specific section on stress, anxiety, worry and fear, and discusses meditation, yoga, and other forms of relaxation all of which are of proven value in the management of dysfunctional stress. Thus, the various principles and techniques of stress management discussed in other articles and books are all in this volume; they are simply ordered differently recognizing that dysfunctional stress is an illness arising when we fail to maintain emotional-spiritual health.

6

The Mind-Body Connection

EMOTIONAL-Spiritual health and physical health are interrelated. They influence one another, and gains or dysfunction in one may encourage gains or dysfunction in the other. This is the "mind-body connection." Acknowledging this relationship and its implications is an important prerequisite to increasing your health competence.

I am a person who carries a lot of tension in the upper back/shoulder/lower neck area. It is my "tension target zone." When I am anxious, one or more muscles in that area tighten up. If I do not stretch them carefully during such periods I will get a spasm in the upper back or a painfully stiff neck, either of which results in days of unpleasant pain. For several years, emotional conflict with a woman important to me would give me a pain in my "tension target zone." Remarkably, however, this relationship tension always caused pain on the *same side* in the *same place*, *exactly* in the same muscle. This phenomenon became laughingly known among some friends as my "woman friend spasm."

This almost trivial story may be meaningful to you. It is a simple illustration of the powerful effects of emotions and tension on the body. Most people have experienced tightness and pain in the upper back and neck. All have experienced emotional tension with a person important to them. This very combination of trigger and target response occurs for some people who are not aware of the relationship between the stress and the discomfort.

Despite innumerable stories like this

one, it is difficult for people to comprehend how frequent, clear, and powerful the mind-body connections are. However, most of us experience these connections every day. For example, nearly everyone has known their heart to beat faster or harder because of excitement or anticipation. It is also common to hear a person say that they have been sweating a great deal in association with increased stress. Most of us increase muscle tension and breathe faster when angry or fearful. Who has not had appetite affected by worry, such as before an exam or important interview?

More dramatic and compelling examples are seen when people become very skilled at controlling certain "autonomic" bodily functions through meditation, imagery, and other kinds of "mind control." Many master yogis can, during meditation, reduce their blood pressure below 50 systolic (the upper number) and their heart rate as low as 30 per minute.

The converse is also true. The body's functions can also affect our emotions and moods. Each of us can probably give personal evidence supporting that statement. Strenuous exercise, for example, can, like worry, definitely decrease one's appetite. Exercise is also justifiably famous for elevating mood and energy levels. Prolonged lack of sleep has such profound effects on the mind that it is used to facilitate criminal interrogation; in extreme instances, it is a form of torture. Finally, even those who have never tried other alternative methods of healing have probably experienced the soothing effects of massage when worried or distraught.

The mind-body connection permeates all of health and illness. A sickness caused largely by poorly managed stress can create definite abnormalities in the body's structure. A disease which appears to have most or all of its roots explained in biological terms (like a severe infection, accident, toxic poisoning, some cancers)

can have powerful impact on one's emotional-spiritual well-being, even to the point of becoming the primary factor in a person's illness. And just as your emotions and spirit may be intimately involved in the genesis of disease, as you get well, the mind may have everything to do with healing. When we examine health and well-being (as contrasted with sickness), the same connections are apparent. Good self-esteem helps a person adopt an exercise program, and the exercise program further enhances self-esteem. A person's willingness to change, be vulnerable, and take risks is related to their emotional-spiritual background and current emotional-spiritual health.

We have already seen that your health beliefs play a significant role in generating the habits and behaviors that determine your risk for heart disease, many cancers, and other problems. These health beliefs are intimately related to your emotional-spiritual health and background, so there may be no such thing as a purely physical or purely emotional-spiritual problem. The workings of body and mind are intricately interwoven. Few days pass that this is not demonstrated clearly for each of us. *Physical and emotional sickness do not exist separately.*

Because the mind-body connection is so basic to health competence, this first chapter in the pathway to emotional-spiritual health is devoted to a further exploration of its nature and impact. "Mind" is a combination of intellectual, emotional, and spiritual functions. Our emotional-spiritual self can affect our body, as when Norman Cousins laughs to defeat his spinal arthritis. On the other hand, our bodies can affect our minds as when a heart attack causes depression. Facts and concepts can also help us heal; if we learn a lot about a particular condition, it may give us confidence and "know how."

Personal health competence includes

the following beliefs about mind-body relationships:

1. Body and mind are interfunctional in the origins and resolution of sickness, disease, and illness. All symptoms, disease, and medical and health problems are caused to some degree by emotional-spiritual factors, and/or have a definite psychological impact on the individual.

For example, some common disorders like high blood pressure and peptic ulcers appear to be caused or influenced by emotional-spiritual determinants: chronic poorly managed stress, unresolved personal and interpersonal tensions (particularly anger), and maladaptation to change or loss. Even the common respiratory infections are not "immune."

An incident in Dr. Kathleen Smith's life further illustrates. Dr. Smith is a young woman in training to become a psychiatrist. She is extremely conscientious about her work and allows little time for pleasure. She reads voluminously, almost all work-connected. Her first two years of psychiatric training were very demanding emotionally and physically. The bill of fare was long hours, nighttime call or training sessions, and very sick, discouraging patients. During one 18-month period she attended three weekend workshops on grieving and loss. She was first a participant, later an instructor. Each time, she became ill. Each time, her symptoms were the same — deep racking cough, profuse running nose, headache, some fever. Each time the illness lasted about ten days and required her to take two to three days off to begin healing.

2. The health care professions, institutions in general, and physicians in particular do not, with few exceptions, practice medicine and health in a way which recognizes mind-body connections in their work. As a result, physicians too often combat disease to the exclusion of healing illness.

3. Every effort that is successful in healing or curing gains some significant part of its effectiveness from the patient's expectation that it will work. This is called the placebo effect.

4. A "medical" problem can also cause psychological difficulties which interfere with its own resolution.

Phil is an example of this last phenomenon. In a bad auto accident he sustained a protruding fracture of the upper bone of the leg. An operation was required, and he was confined to the hospital for ten days. He worried a lot about not being able to work and feared he might lose his job. He remained silent, becoming severely depressed. This interfered significantly with physical therapy and other efforts which were an important part of his rehabilitation. His progress was slow.

One day as the physical therapist was over-enthusiastically encouraging him, he broke down in tearful frustration. He told her his concerns. She subsequently communicated them to the nursing staff who called his employer. This man, though busy, visited Phil in the hospital. He spent some time and effort reassuring Phil that his job was secure. Even given some permanent change in Phil's physical capabilities, the boss said they would find a way of modifying his job so that he could make a full contribution.

A second visit a few days later was accompanied by the same reassurances. Thereafter, Phil's depression lifted and his rehabilitation progressed rapidly. He was able to return to work at his old job.

The body-mind connection also operates in two common fatal diseases, coronary artery disease, which causes most heart attacks, and cancer.

CORONARY ARTERY DISEASE (HEART ATTACK) AND HYPERTENSION (HIGH BLOOD PRESSURE)

A number of factors, called risk factors, increase the likelihood that a person will develop significant coronary artery disease. A person who has a risk factor is said to be at increased *risk* for heart disease. High blood pressure or hypertension is one of the most serious risk factors for heart disease.

The relationship of stress to blood pressure is well established. Acute stress can produce sudden rises in blood pressure, and chronic stress is a crucial — if not the most important — factor in causing hypertension or chronic high blood pressure. Thus, stress can increase the likelihood that a person will get coronary artery disease through its affect on the blood pressure.

People can also increase their stress-related risk for heart attack more directly, that is without the effect of high blood pressure. The "type A" personalities described by Friedman[1] are more prone to heart attack than their "type B" counterparts. This type A personality has two salient characteristics. One is an exaggerated awareness of and reaction to time pressure — a self-imposed need to constantly set and meet deadlines. The other is competitiveness. Type A people are intensely competitive at work, at home, and even in their leisure. This combination of characteristics has been nicknamed "hurry sickness." Type As also judge their accomplishments primarily in terms of numbers — the number of reports they produce, the amount of their salary, the number of miles they run, scores on tests, and grades in school. Their security rests primarily on the quantity of achievement, not necessarily on quality. In contrast, type B people are significantly less likely to become "victims" of heart disease. They are more relaxed, less competitive, and do not have a continuous sense of time urgency. Interestingly, they are *not* less successful!

Emotional stress, therefore, can increase a person's risk for heart attack both

by raising blood pressure and by the need of some people to respond to stress in a type A way.

CANCER

There is probably no disorder more widely feared than cancer. Most people think and talk of cancer as a mystery over which an individual has no control. Nowhere in medicine is the "victim" mentality more pronounced, i.e., "poor John, he has cancer." However, recent evidence suggests that such attitudes may not be entirely justified. In fact, they may be counterproductive in terms of cancer prevention and treatment.

Carl and Stephanie Simonton[2] speak of a psychological process which frequently precedes cancer. It distinguishes those who do from those who don't get cancer; the following elements may or may not all be evident in the same person:

1. Childhood experiences lead to decisions to be a certain kind of person, e.g., since my father hits my mother I will always be gentle and not "get angry." "Or some children make an early decision that they are responsible for the feelings of other people, and whenever other people are unhappy or sad . . . it's their responsibility to help them feel better."

2. A "cluster" of stressful life events occur in the ten-year period before the cancer appears. They threaten personal identity: e.g., a student graduates from college, leaves the student role, and must earn his own living; a homemaker who has "existed" to support her husband's career and raise their children finds the children gone from home and her husband suddenly dead from a heart attack.

3. One or more of these events create a problem difficult or impossible for the

1. M. Friedman, *Type A Behavior and Your Heart* (New York: Alfred Knopf, 1974).

2. Carl Simonton and Stephanie Simonton. *Getting Well Again* (New York: Bantam Books, 1978).

person to deal with because of the rules he/she has set up in early life. For example, the woman cited above may have decided in early life that she would be passive and meek like her mother, since she herself had suffered from her father's aggression. Now that her husband is dead and children gone, she finds it difficult to become aggressive enough to successfully find a good job.

4. As a result, the individual now sees no way to change the rules about how he must act and consequently feels trapped and helpless — the victim mentality of "Life is acting upon me" (not they upon their lives).

5. The individual becomes static, unchanging, and rigid. Although externally the individual may seem to be coping well, internally life holds no meaning. Serious illness then represents a solution or postponement to the problem.

Not only have the Simontons identified this mind-body process leading up to the development of cancer, they have also had success in slowing the progress of terminal cancer by helping people reverse these "hangups" and attitudes and by having them actively and repetitively visualize their cellular defense mechanisms against cancer as becoming more active and aggressive. Through such guided visualizations, psychotherapy, strategies designed to overcome communication blocks, and awakening spirituality, they have obtained remarkable improvement in the length and quality of life for many of their cancer patients. "They are victims no longer."

THE PLACEBO EFFECT

The placebo effect is one of the best studied and most compelling illustrations of the body-mind connection. It is the cura-

tive or healing change derived from the positive expectations of the patient that the treatment will work. Many experiments have been conducted in which patients receiving sugar pills have gotten well with almost the same frequency and efficiency as those who received real medicine. This is due to the placebo effects. It is so significant, in fact, that the effects of many new drugs are now determined in one group of patients and compared with those of a sugar pill or other inert substance in a comparable group of patients.

The patient's positive expectations are created for the most part by a person's physician or other health provider, or by the person's own belief in doctors or medications. An inert medication (like a sugar pill) often produces the desired effect if the person receiving the medication *believes* it will work. The effect also operates when a health provider confidently creates positive expectations about a *real* medication. In other words, part of the beneficial effect of real pills or injections is derived from the person's confidence that the medicine will have the desired effect (see Figure 6–1).

It is likely that the positive effects of both orthodox medical practices and folk healers have depended partly on the placebo effect. We know, for example, that the practice of bloodletting could have had no rational benefit for most problems. Yet it seemed helpful in some cases. Both physicians and patients believed it would work!

An even more dramatic example has been observed in patients for whom a particular surgical procedure on the chest wall for coronary artery disease seemed indicated. The procedure involved tying off an arterial supply in the chest wall which, it was reasoned, resulted in more blood for the heart. In two different studies patients were randomly divided into two groups as their indications for

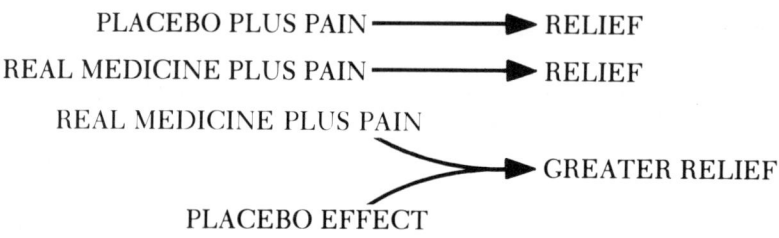

FIGURE 6-1   Expectations and the Placebo Effect

surgery became apparent. One group had the full operation. The other group simply had their chest wall incised in the same way, but the internal mammary arteries were not tied off. Subsequently, both groups improved their symptoms and by comparable amounts!

Thus, the placebo effect is major evidence of the power that the mind can have upon the body in the healing process. When our faith in our own healing powers and those of non-medication alternatives is as strong as our belief in medications, their potential to help us is greatly enhanced.

HEALTH PROFESSIONALS AND THE MIND-BODY CONNECTION

Belief in the interrelations of body and mind with respect to health and illness is not new. Credence for a synergistic view has existed since the days of medical antiquity. Numerous contemporary folk and psychic healers utilize the relationship with notable success. In the last forty years, however, there has been a sharp and lamentable decline in the extent to which body-mind connections are attended to in the "formal" practice of medicine and in the education of health professionals. The widespread and frequent use of valium and other tranquilizers, however, suggests that many practicing physicians acknowledge it.

The management of headache is a case in point. Almost everyone has headaches. Most of us respond to aspirin, and we think nothing about it. Here is a somewhat different story.

Sharon's headaches began on an occasional basis but soon occurred almost every day. They involved both sides of her head. The pain was dull, moderate in severity, and very tenacious and steady, often becoming a disturbing preoccupation. The headaches were more likely to occur as the day progressed, and although helped by aspirin, they were never completely relieved.

Sharon went to her physician. After a short period of questioning and a brief examination he ordered "tests." In the next two weeks she had skull X-rays, an electroencephalogram (brain wave), a brain scan, blood tests, urinalysis, and tests for her thyroid. Cost of the tests and more visits to her physician was almost $550.00. "Nothing" was found. The headaches remained unchanged, despite a prescription for valium. Finally, on her own, Sharon went to see a psychotherapist. She suspected that the headache might be more related to certain tensions at work or the concern that her eldest son was taking drugs. The therapist probed carefully into some of these possibilities. She asked simple questions. "Has anything changed in your life lately?" And later, "Well, there are certainly reasons for tension in your life at home, how about at work?" She was able to encourage Sharon to disclose and discuss her concerns at greater length. Together they worked out ways she might resolve the difficulties directly rather than worrying about them and doing nothing. Sharon's headaches improved almost immediately. Within a few weeks they were gone.

Sharon's first physician was either unaware or unwilling to acknowledge the potential significance of the mind-body connection in her case. Time and money were wasted. Healing was delayed.

In the education of health professionals, body-mind considerations, when presented at all, are overshadowed by material on normal structure, function, and disease that students are required to learn. Few leave training ready or able to completely attend to the intricate, often delicate, and carefully concealed body-mind connections. This lack of sufficient awareness and attention to the body-mind association among health practitioners, particularly physicians, partly explains, I believe, the narrow, technical approach of most medical professionals.

The lack of attention to the body-mind connection by medical schools and specialty training programs has been reinforced by the rapid technologic and scientific advances in medicine, and by methods of payment, which reward skill in doing procedures, far more than time spent talking to and caring for patients. A specialist in gastrointestinal disease can earn $200 in 20 minutes by doing a gastroscopic exam of the stomach. If, as commonly occurs, the problem is one that embodies important psychological factors, the same physician is able to bill only a few dollars for additional time spent talking with the patient. This results in extreme emphasis on the body in terms of symptoms, disease, and injury. To be sure, great attention and resources are devoted to mental disorders, but these services are functionally and organizationally disconnected from "body medicine."

Imagine yourself with a certain disorder, let's say a sore throat with fever, which causes you to go to bed, lose time from work or school and feel depressed. You begin to realize that you are uncomfortable, tired, and feverish. Also, you experience uselessness, helplessness, and worry about missing school, or work, or both, and how you will make them up. You may feel lonely if your friends are all at work or school. This combination of symptoms and their impact constitute *illness*, as contrasted with the sore throat and fever considered in isolation, which is your *disease*.

Disease is defined as an alteration in the structure or function of an organ or organ system (in the example above, the sore throat). The existence of a person in, around, and involved with the disease is not necessary. *Illness*, on the other hand, encompasses the often major, even overwhelming, contribution of emotional, social, and economic factors to the *origin, perpetuation, and impact* of the problem on the patient. The latter can include helplessness, a loss of omnipotence, unusual dependency on others, and a sense of disconnectedness from the rest of the world. More specific items, such as worries about finances, the children's well-being, or why Sally hasn't come to see me today, may also be of major concern (see Figure 6-2).

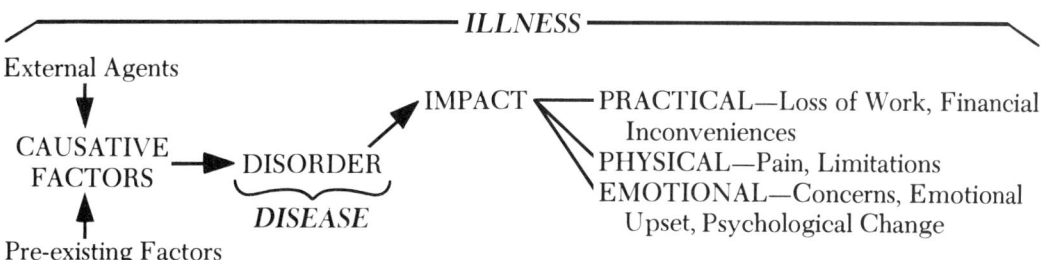

FIGURE 6-2.

Eric Cassell, in *The Healer's Art*,[3] has carefully distinguished disease and illness. He has also defined *curing* as the process of resolving disease (if the doctor is successful!) and *healing* as the process that manages, ameliorates, and disperses the illness:

When examining someone who is ill, every physician is so accustomed to looking for the causative disease that the cause of illness is inevitably confused with the phenomenon of illness itself. But the illness and the disease must really be quite separate entities, since sick people have certain characteristics in common and behave in certain similar ways regardless of whether they are sick with pneumonia or have a fractured leg. Thus it seemed obvious that making the distinction between illness and disease could be extremely useful in helping me understand patients and the role of doctors.

I then realized that there must be a similar distinction between healing and curing. If the sick person indeed presents two distinct aspects of his sickness — the illness and the disease that caused it — the doctor must respond with two separate functions, no matter how closely connected they may be or how the curing function may conceal the healing function. To the doctor who does not distinguish between illness and disease, making a patient with pneumonia better means curing the pneumonia — killing the bacteria, bringing down his fever, enabling him to breathe more easily. Indeed, if the doctor does not do those things, it will be bad news for the patient. But there are other aspects of the illness that the doctor may ignore: the patient may be frightened about what is happening in his body; he may feel cut off from his family and his friends; and he may find himself painfully dependent on other people. Handling those aspects of the patient's pneumonia is also part of the doctor's job, a part of his healing function that can be viewed as entirely separate from his function in curing the pneumonia, even if, in practice, the two functions are interrelated.

3. Eric Cassell, *The Healer's Art* (New York: Penguin Books, 1979) pp. 16, 17. Grateful acknowledgment is made to Eric Cassell and Penguin Books for permission to reprint a passage from *The Healer's Art.*

The important point to understand is that illness is more than just disease or disorder alone — often a lot more. Illness exists because of body-mind connections. Since few physicians are well trained to recognize and deal with body-mind connections, illness is usually neglected. The disorder is cared for but not its impact; the disease is cured, but the illness is not healed.

Efforts toward health and the treatment of medical disorders are incomplete unless the mind-body connection is acknowledged and incorporated into the approach. In order to maximize the full potential of patient appraisal and treatment, both the health provider and the client need to approach problems as interactive products of both body and mind.

In summary, the body and mind essentially work as one. A physical problem does not exist without emotional-spiritual impact. Emotional illness often has associated physical symptoms (e.g., sleeping poorly when depressed). Healing either the illnesses we call emotional or those we call physical is greatly facilitated by belief in our own power to heal ourselves and faith in other therapies that are used. People who are healthy in the emotional-spiritual realm have a head start on health and health competence. The next chapter will begin to define emotional-spiritual health.

RESOURCES CHAPTER 6

Cassell, E.J. *The Healer's Art. A New Approach to the Doctor-Patient Relationship.* New York: Penguin Books, 1976. A very important statement. It provides understanding of the basic tensions between doctor and patient and offers hope for solutions.

Jaffé, Q.T. *Healing From Within.* New York: Knopf, 1980. This is a wellness workbook for those who are ill. An important statement that also furnishes the skills and strategies for optimizing and actively participating in recovery.

Peck, M.S. *The Road Less Traveled*. New York: Touchstone, Simon and Schuster, 1978. A compelling and very useful treatise on personal growth which discusses the parts played by discipline, love, and grace in that process. Few books of this kind are as useful.

Pelletier, K. *Mind As Healer, Mind As Slayer*. New York: Delta/Dell, 1977. A scholarly, detailed up-to-date treatise on the complexities of mind-body relationships. Well referenced.

Simonton, O.C., Matthews-Simonton, S., Creighton, J.S. *Getting Well Again*. New York: Bantam Books, 1978. How the authors use the mind-body connection to help people cope with and progress against cancer.

7

Individual Emotional-Spiritual Health

GAINING the confidence and skills to take care of one's emotional and spiritual needs in healthy, loving, non-manipulative ways is the task of emotional-spiritual health competence. It is not easy, because for the awakened person each life situation is a new challenge and place to grow. Each step along the path brings you closer to your true self, allows you to relate more closely to other people, and may bring external gains as well. Except perhaps for saints, however, the job is never finished.

ESSAY: ACTIVE SPIRITUALITY

When I first sat down to write about spirituality and spiritual wellness, I was not sure how to begin. Not many years ago I would not have included this emphasis at all. Now it seems essential. This book would be incomplete without major attention to spirituality and what I call emotional-spiritual health. Why is this? What has changed for me in that time?

As an adolescent, I remember intermittent awareness of a higher power, a force spirit or energy that was "outside" me yet part of me, infinite yet accessible. The awareness was most likely to occur when I was in the mountains or in some other relatively untouched or uninhabited place: at night under the stars or skiing pell-mell down a slope.

I have never joined a formal religion and although my experience with church has been brief and unsustained, it was significant. While in high school I attended a Methodist church three times a month during the winter season so that I could qualify to play on their basketball team. Later, my first several months in college were the unhappiest, loneliest, and most frightening of my life. During that time I went to bed every night convinced I would die before morning. Through fear, I attended the non-denominational chapel on the campus every Sunday. It was a great comfort; I am sure it helped me survive the experience and even to do well in school. Finally, in the months before my marriage and for a few years thereafter, I attended Catholic mass occasionally with my wife and children, who were Catholic. Then sometimes I was again aware of some power greater than myself.

From about the age of 30 until I was 51 or 52, I was essentially bankrupt spiritually — not because I didn't attend church, but because my sense and acknowledgment of a power greater than myself was non-existent. The only exception to that occurred when I was on Henry Island. Somehow, there, I often felt that everything was part of a larger whole over which I had no real control. I felt like a small unit in an interconnected human and mystical world.

My friend John defines someone as spiritual if they are able to imagine the existence of some force, power, or being that connects with them to provide guidance, nurturing, or protection. In this sense, the spirit is our mystical part, the unknown, the magical. For most people, he feels, this power is a friendly one that has influence over them, provides them with energy, or does some combination of these things. His way of thinking about it makes sense to me, but it is also incomplete, because it doesn't explicitly include an additional strong sense that I experience from people who are spiritual. That sense is that they are basically loving: they come from a space that is loving, peaceful, and often joyful.

It is also important to say what I think

spirituality is not. It is not necessarily a belief in God. It is not membership in a formal religion. I don't believe that membership in or observance of the rituals of an organized religion necessarily has much to do with being spiritual; some of the most spiritual people I know have never belonged to an organized religion. It is not ritualistic behavior; it is not adherence to a specific set of dogma or beliefs of some religion or sect. It does not, on the other hand, exclude any of these things, and certainly they are all compatible with an active and healthful spirituality.

Perhaps, more than anything else, spirituality is the acknowledgment or imagination that some force, power, or being exists, which supercedes all of us, but particularly oneself — we are not our own higher power. I believe this power connects me to all other human beings. In that sense, we are all spiritual. For some that higher power is a group of people from whom they take nurturing and sustenance. For others, it is simply Love. For most, it is God. Perhaps they are all the same.

My own emotional-spiritual growth has been nourished and sustained from a number of important sources. One has been the love of my family and friends. Even in my worst times, sometimes unknowingly, they encouraged me to live rather than die. I have been in individual therapy four different times for a total of about three years. This has given me support and understanding, which have greatly assisted my "growing work." I have belonged to support groups. The most important one, though not a formal religion, has a very spiritual program. It has helped me recognize the unity of emotional and spiritual health. Of major importance, I have advised, guided, listened to, and supported family members, friends, students, and patients in their journey toward greater emotional-spiritual health. This has helped me as much or more than it has them.

Certain books have also been highly important in shaping my thinking and faith. *The Prophet* has been the most enduring of these. Gibran's words about self-knowledge speak to the essence of emotional-spiritual health:

> But let there be no scales to weigh your unknown treasures:
> And seek not the depths of your knowledge with staff or sounding line.
> For self is a sea boundless and measureless.
> Say not, "I have found the truth," but rather, "I have found a truth."
> Say not, "I have found the path of the soul." Say rather,
> "I have met the soul walking upon my path."[1]

Actualizations, a small book by Stuart Emory, makes good common sense (which is what a lot of emotional-spiritual health is about). Recent books by Hugh Prather (especially *The Quiet Answer*) provide me with endless challenge. Peck's *The Road Less Traveled* is a moving and lucid statement about mental health, growth, love, and guidance. It is a book to return to often. *A Way of Life* by William Osler, influenced me strongly to try and live one day at a time or (as Osler, calls them) in "day-tight compartments."

Though not always so, my emotional-spiritual health is good now. From a time when I was spiritually bankrupt, angry, despairing, sometimes suicidal, I strive now to be honest, emotionally vulnerable, spiritually energetic, open to criticism and suggestions for change. My main way is loving and peaceful—I am growing.

Finally, I am a good coach. Good

coaches are seldom former champions and are never perfect. This chapter and following ones are my effort to advise and coach you through an assessment of your own emotional-spiritual health and a consideration of the choices and changes available. It feels good to be doing this.

ESSAY: FEELINGS IN GENERAL, ANGER IN PARTICULAR

When I was a child I was confused about feelings. It seemed as though my parents were always telling me (directly or indirectly) how to feel. I frequently hear other parents doing that. It is probably the biggest single problem with parents. They can't resist the compulsion to tell their kids how to feel, and they are not always direct about it. In fact, if I told someone, "you spend a lot of time telling your kid what to feel and what not to feel," or "you're usurping your kid's feelings," they'd get hurt, angry, or deny it.

But it's true. For example, a kid falls down, skins his knee, and starts to cry. The parent says, "That doesn't hurt; you can stop crying now." Or if the child feels frustration or anger at someone and lets it out, the dad says, "Now you shouldn't be angry at Mrs. so-and-so. I want you to go right back there and apologize." These reactions tell the child not to have feelings and not to express them. Telling people not to have feelings takes away something that is theirs.

The fact is that feelings just *are*, and they are *yours*. Like blood pressure, pulse rate, skin color, and other bodily functions, feelings *are*, too. They are an important indicator of your emotional state, just the way your pulse or blood pressure or respiratory rate are indicators of your physical state. Feelings are tricky; whether we acknowledge it or not, we all work from them. For this reason they need to be acknowledged and dealt with honestly.

Telling people to feel or not to feel a

1. Kahlil Gibran, *The Prophet* (New York: Alfred Knopf, 1966). Grateful acknowledgement is made to Alfred A. Knopf for permission to reprint material from *The Prophet* by Kahlil Gibran.

certain way will cause suppression, repression, or distortion of emotions. Many times a feeling stimulates old patterns of behavior — turns on that same old tape that it has for years. I feel rejected, I withdraw, and then I am alone. This gets us in the same trouble over and over again. To learn from a feeling we must first experience it. Sadness may be an important indication of an unprocessed loss or an unfulfilled need, but unless we experience it we can never learn that.

Anger is probably the most mismanaged emotion in our culture. Although it is more acceptable for men to get angry than women, neither sex handles anger well. Men too often use it as a verbal weapon or as an excuse to be physically abusive or manipulative. Women are more likely not to express it at all. Many do not feel it or turn it back in on themselves, becoming passive or depressed. In groups, it is not uncommon for a woman to say, after a number of meetings, that they didn't even *recognize* the feeling of anger until they had been in the group for a while. They had repressed the feeling so thoroughly it wasn't apparent to them even when it was stimulated.

One common result of mismanaged anger is that anger at one person may come out against another. This is called displaced anger. As a young boy, I expressed tremendous anger on the tennis court. All the anger I felt I shouldn't express at other times came out on the court, released by some little mistake or the loss of one point.

In a way, it is understandable that we are taught to "stuff" our anger. Terrible things happen as a result of anger. Violence is one. But that's the rub. Violence occurs when a person builds up anger over a period of time without processing or expressing it as it occurs. Tolerance is eventually exceeded, the pressure valve blows, and the person erupts, becoming verbally or physically abusive.

Parents who have been on the receiving end of such eruptive anger are uncomfortable with anger in their children and set about suppressing it by ordering their children, in essence, not to feel it. Unfortunately, this sets the stage for the child to become an eruptor also or to develop and harbor long-term resentments, another common consequence of "stuffing it."

Healthy people learn to express their anger in a non-harmful manner. One way is to tell the object of your anger, in an even voice, that they have made you angry and why. For example, "The job was supposed to be done two days ago, and it's not. I'm angry about that." This requires separating the expression of anger from judgment about the person's worth, their "badness" or "goodness." What you didn't like and got angry at was what they did (or didn't do). You can still like them or love them (or both). "Johnny," said his mother, "I love you very much but I don't like it when you trample mud on my carpets."

Sometimes when you feel intense anger or if the object of your anger is particularly fragile, it is better to ventilate your anger before, or instead of, expressing it to the person. One of the best ways to do this is to simply sit down and write about it.

A number of other things work for me, and I do all of them alone. One is to pound on pillows while yelling "at" the person I'm angry at. Some people like to start in a subdued tone, build up to a frenzy, and then taper off with a repetitive phrase like, "I'm angry but I love you." Another strategy is go for a drive and yell out all the things, including judgments, that you want to say. Gradually, as you repeat them the anger will dissipate. Another of my favorite coping methods is to yell as I run. Finally, try backing off from the circumstances which aroused the anger and take care of yourself for a while. Do something you want to do for yourself. Later return to the task of resolving your anger. You will have put it in much better perspective.

ESSAY: LIVING IN "DAY-TIGHT" COMPARTMENTS OR ONE DAY AT A TIME

As a young boy I can remember living in the future a lot: wishing my birthday or Christmas or vacation would come. Some days I would lie around doing nothing but wishing that the next of those great events would come. Early in medical school I was having difficulty coping with the enormous amount of material we had to learn. Medicine as a career seemed more distant than ever — I was doing a lot of looking ahead and some wistful looking back.

One day, I came across a little book by William Osler called *A Way of Life*. Osler was one of the famous quartet of physicians at Johns Hopkins Medical School in the early 1900's. He was widely acclaimed for his knowledge, his original investigations, and his compassion. The book had particular meaning to me because my grandfather, a physician, had been Osler's first medical resident at Hopkins.

A Way of Life intrigued me. It argued for living each day by focusing attention and energy on the issues, problems, and joys of that day. The past was considered history, the future as a mystery, a time which would take care of itself by living in "day-tight compartments," as Osler called them. Partly because of my need for stability, partly because of Osler's powerful style, I was compelled to try this "way of life." I did so for some time, not perfectly and not with consistency (because it is not easy), but diligently enough to make a significant difference for me. I was happier, less scattered, able to work more effectively, and able to more fully enjoy my free time.

After a year or so, I gradually slipped away from living one day at a time. I never tried it again consistently until 30 years later. Then, as part of my personal program for health competence, I again adopted the day at a time philosophy and way of life. It is probably the single most valuable tool I have to live by. For me, it works well. I don't always remember to practice it, but when I do, each moment is enriched. Time is not lost in belaboring the mistakes of the past or wishing for some wonderful future. It is profoundly true that this moment is all we really have — it pays to make the most of it.

I think many emotionally well people live in day-tight compartments. They may not have a phrase to describe it, but they *live* the philosophy. They may use past mistakes to make informed decisions in the present, but they don't wallow around in those mistakes, blaming, resenting, and feeling guilty. Neither are past successes used as an emotional shot in the arm for today. Although they plan ahead to the extent necessary, they don't "wish" ahead (as I did with my birthdays). They don't "live for the day when;" they simply live today.

THE EMOTIONALLY WELL PERSON

Several years ago I got tired of reading about neuroses and maladjustment and manipulation and other things we consider unhealthy. I began to wonder what was emotionally *healthy*. Was it just the absence of the unhealthy traits or something more than that? Moreover, I was much more interested in what the average, non-medically oriented layperson thought than psychiatrists and other mental health workers. So I began asking various groups I worked with to develop definitions. However, before looking at what they did, why don't you try it? Simply write in your notebook what you believe are the most important characteristics of the emotionally healthy person (I was not at that time using the term emotional-spiritual health, which I now prefer).

Now look at Table 7-1. It represents a group opinion compiled by a method which permitted everyone to prioritize not just their own items but those of their classmates as well. The language is that of the group.

I want to emphasize several aspects of this chart. First, the global characteristic "feels good about self" was *always* chosen and was first on two-thirds of the lists. In the words of Pelletier[2] ". . . You are healthy when you are most yourself . . . do anything that gives you a sense of enthusiasm and joy — and be yourself." And, it could be added, esteem yourself.

Second, the emotionally well person "accepts the responsibility and power for life's choices." This was selected by two-thirds of the group. This reflects the central importance of self-responsibility ("ownership") in Personal Health Competence.

Third, it is clear that dealing effectively with feelings is important: "can laugh at oneself," "communicates feelings

2. Kenneth Pelletier, *Mind is Healer, Mind is Slayer* (New York: Delta/Dell, 1977).

openly and honestly," "handles strong feelings constructively," and "puts things in perspective" are all items which support this as a basic requirement.

Fourth, the importance of discriminating between environments (the group meant the human environment) that are nurturing and non-nurturing was clear. While it is often difficult to make choices about one's natural environment because of financial constraints and job commitments, it *is* usually possible to make choices about one's circle of acquaintances and friends, i.e., the personal environment.

Finally, while several of these items have spiritual implications (feels good about self, can laugh at oneself, giving of time and talents for others), none describes traits which are explicitly spiritual. At the time, I was asking for a definition of "emotional health" not "emotional-spiritual health," which probably explains this. Since that time, it is obvious to me that active spirituality is an essential aspect of emotional-spiritual health.

THE PROCESS OF EMOTIONAL-SPIRITUAL HEALTH COMPETENCE

My own experience, observations, and work lead me to describe an overall process and propose a set of skills for

TABLE 7–1 **A Group Definition of the Emotionally Well Person.**

Priority	Characteristic
1	Feels good about self
2	Gladly accepts the responsibility and power for life's choices (and is happy with the power)
	Discriminates nurturing and non-nurturing environment and chooses former
3	Can laugh at oneself
	Communicates feelings openly and honestly
	Handles strong feelings constructively
	Handles stress constructively
	Puts things in perspective
4	Ability to ascribe worth to others
	Appreciates positives in environment
	Sees self as others do
	Giving of time and talents for others

emotional-spiritual health, which embody the factors just emphasized and add other characteristics as well.

A person's emotional-spiritual health can be characterized by a predominant energy state or spirit in which most behavior is carried out. For a given individual, this dominant spirit lies somewhere along the continuum shown in Figure 7-1. With emotional-spiritual growth, the predominant spirit is characterized less and less by anger, conflict, and fear and more and more by love, peace, and joy.

People differ in the quality of the energy with which they usually perceive and act. Some seem to live mainly from a place of love, peace, and joy. Those energies are at once their outlook and their purpose. Any situation which is uncertain in temperament is first seen as peaceful, and their approach to it reflects that. They expect most situations to produce positive outcomes, and they look for that. Though well able to experience and express anger, their basic spirit is not angry. They know misfortune, and they suffer, but they grow as well. They are not strangers to fear, especially realistic fear, but transcend it in much of their daily toil.

At the other extreme are those who deal mainly from anger, conflict, and fear. That is their dominant spirit. In most situations they find or create anger, fear, and suspicion. In the extreme, they experience whatever others do as an attack and interpret the proceedings in that light. They expect most situations to produce a negative outcome.

Probably a minority of people operate predominately near one end of this continuum or the other. Most are in between. These "in-betweeners" can come from either of the two extreme positions in certain circumstances, but most of the time they operate from some middle ground which might be characterized as manipulative, ambivalent, and anxious.

Some time ago, I shared with another person two days of positive feelings and good communication. The visit was followed by several phone calls in the same spirit. Then it became impossible for me to reach her. For four weeks I left unanswered messages on an answering machine. Then I sent a mailgram which expressed concern for the person's well-being. In case something had happened to her (which seemed a genuine possibility at this point), I addressed it not only to the person herself but to the other people she lived with. A few days later she called me. She was very angry. She said that my calls and mailgram were manipulative and coercive, and that she had been troubled and hadn't wanted to talk to me. Her reasons for isolation seemed reasonable. The point is she interpreted my actions as hostile, manipulative, and not caring—and reacted from an angry space. For my part, I operated more from anxiety than from peace and love. The mailgram was definitely intended to get a response from her and in that sense was manipulative. If I had been entirely loving, I would have probably left her completely alone. If she had been more loving, she would have seen my concern as an expression of caring.

So, as people grow in emotional-spiritual health, their basic spirit is less angry, conflicted, and fearful, and more loving, peaceful, and joyful. Most impor-

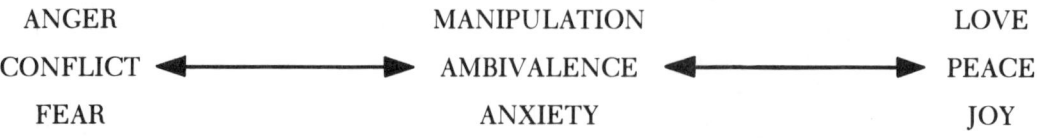

ANGER	MANIPULATION	LOVE
CONFLICT ⟷	AMBIVALENCE ⟷	PEACE
FEAR	ANXIETY	JOY

FIGURE 7-1   The Continuum of Emotional-Spiritual Health.

tantly, *emotional-spiritual health is the process of moving along the continuum:* it is not a matter of reaching the loving end and coming to a stop. No one ever reaches the end — there is always farther to go. We may falter at times and not move (this is being stuck) for weeks or even months, but eventually as we begin to move again our emotional-spiritual health improves. A person whose spirit is still basically angry and fearful but who is working to change, can be healthier than one whose spirit is basically manipulative and anxious but who is also stuck. An acquaintance of mine said, "I can't just jump to the top of a mountain and stay there, I must climb."

The relationship of this growing process to our feelings, particularly anger, is critical. Many of us who grew up in middle-class America where anger is so inhibited or in lower-class America where there is so much to be angry about must emerge through an angry period before we can be peaceful. This has certainly been true of me. For many years, even as I began growing in emotional health, I was rooted in anger, conflict, and fear. I needed to work through that (often slow work) before my spirit changed to become more loving, peaceful, and joyful. Perhaps saints are people who actually arrive at the loving end of this continuum and stay there. The rest of us, even the emotionally healthiest, will continue to have times when we come from an angry or manipulative stance, but as we grow in emotional health, those times will occur less often and be shorter in duration.

An individual's progress along the continuum of emotional-spiritual health depends on several important things. The presence of healthy or relatively healthy people to serve as models is one. Access (including financial access) to education and counseling is another. Acceptance of self-responsibility is basic to the growth

process, but for many people, questions of survival and acceptance have greater immediacy than a priority for growth in emotional-spiritual health. Those who suffer economic poverty, racial injustice, or other disadvantages often cannot make the task of improving their emotional-spiritual health an explicit issue because they are overwhelmed by matters of survival — food, housing, education, and violence. To grow, they must often move against subculture and peer-group values which nourish crime, drug abuse, and despair. This does not mean that disadvantaged people cannot grow in emotional-spiritual health. Many, miraculously, can and do. But it is difficult, sometimes too difficult, until basic needs are met. Those of us who do not have those disadvantages are privileged in being able to see and give high priority to our growth.

BEHAVIORS (SKILLS) CHARACTERISTIC OF EMOTIONAL-SPIRITUAL HEALTH

Emotionally healthy people behave in certain ways to increase their inner peace, move into greater harmony with others, and do more productive work. Each healthy person probably exerts a few of these traits most of the time, and some of them part of the time. As they progress, they behave more and more in these ways. The traits are discussed here in an approximate order of importance.

Have a loving relationship with yourself. This means self-esteem ("feel good about self") and more. It is a self-esteem*ing* thing. Take care of yourself in a variety of ways (exercise, vacation, spiritual enrichment, play, time to yourself, laughter) and regard this as a top priority. Don't put yourself down, even in small ways (see essay on Put-Downs in the next chapter). Forgive yourself your mistakes and weaknesses. Be satisfied with progress — you'll never be perfect.

Accept deeply the responsibility for yourself—who and what you are. This requires a willingness to be both involved and accountable. It requires an ability to accurately assess and acknowledge your own strengths and weaknesses, a certain ease with discovering and admitting mistakes, and the strength to acknowledge them. Rather than blame others when something goes amiss, look for your contribution to the difficulty and work to remedy that. You are not a victim but an activated person.

Acknowledge feelings of all kinds as important indicators of your emotional state. Most of us have more mechanisms for covering up feelings than for dealing with them. The emotionally healthy strive to be aware of their feelings, even difficult ones. State and process your feelings in ways that are generally productive, rather than destructive. This does not mean that you can't be assertive or vehement.

Discipline yourself. Discipline is an essential tool for personal effectiveness and growth. Peck in *The Road Less Traveled* gives a clear and very helpful discussion of discipline. He describes four kinds. The first is that of *taking responsibility*, which has already been discussed. Another is *delaying gratification*. This is a process of scheduling your labor and your play so as to get the tough tasks done and enhance the pleasure in life. Doing homework before watching television at night is an example. *Openness to challenge* is a third. Simply, this is the ability to listen to criticism, honestly assess the value of the comments, and then to improve. More profoundly, it involves a willingness to have your deepest values and most ingrained behaviors challenged without reflexively defending yourself or backing away. Finally, there is *dedication to truth*, or honesty. This starts with being truthful and behaving in honest ways. This includes honest appraisal of

yourself and the way you are and things are. This is the process of distinguishing reality from illusion.

Turn on and nurture your spirituality. This may mean actively imagining or fantasizing about God or some other power higher than yourself. Emotionally healthy people believe there is some kind of universal energy available to support all of us. It may indeed *be* all of us—it may be a power that can come from within each of us. It may be a mystical power (most commonly referred to in this country as God). They maintain regular contact with that higher power through prayer, meditation, or conversations throughout the day.

Have allies. We all need emotional support and physical contact from others. The most ardent of these people provide you unwavering support, affirmation, and enhancement. Entrust these allies with your deepest secrets, disclose your vulnerabilities, knowing that you are safe and that you will not be maligned or put down. If you are making a change in your life, first trust allies with the news. You know they will support you.

Be loving. A genuine capacity to love is always evident in healthy people. Love here is defined as the will or the *commitment* to extend yourself for the purpose of nurturing your own or another's emotional-spiritual growth. This implies that love of self and love of others go hand-in-hand. The words "will" and "commitment" indicate action, not just desire. Many people want to love others, but don't do it. Defined as it is above, it is important to recognize that love requires work and often courage as well. It is not necessary to even like a person that you are loving. If you are working to nurture and encourage someone's growth, you are loving them. Loving can be as simple as cooking a meal for your children or as intense as a long-term commitment to an intimate partnership. You cannot be healthy as an individual without loving others.

Make important decisions with your whole being: intellect, feelings, and your spirit. Unless urgency is required, take time to decide and spend a lot of that time watching and listening to yourself and others. Important decisions will then be congruent with your values and goals as well as with your intellectual view of the problem. Do not spend a lot of time intellectually tabulating the pros and cons. That data can be used, of course, but it is best integrated rather than used in isolation.

Acknowledge your lack of perfection. Be open to criticism and fully accepting of the fact that you make mistakes, that you can and will be wrong, that there may often be a better way than the one you are invested in. Emotionally well people seem to be more invested in changing and growing than in anything else.

Use emotional difficulties and crises as lessons and stimuli for growth. We can grow and heal and learn from emotional problems as well as physical ones. This truth is appreciated by the emotionally well, and they are rather consistent in their ability to turn seeming adversity into a learning experience (though they often do this unconsciously). They are much less likely than most of us to become depressed in the face of emotional trauma and much more likely to profit from it in the long run. To be well, don't indulge in the illusion that you can continue to do things the same way and expect different outcomes.

Don't expect constant progress. Run your mind along a piece of bamboo — it is a series of smooth sections interrupted at regular intervals by bumps and splicings. If the sections were irregularly spaced that piece of bamboo would be a good metaphor for a person's growth pattern: a series of active phases punctuated by pauses, quiescent times, even periods of being stuck.

Get out of yourself. A certain amount of introspection is vital to growth, experiencing one's feelings is essential, and solitude can be an important stimulus to growth. However, it is extremely important not to get enmeshed in constant self-analysis, self-pity, rationalization, and self-justification. "Getting out of yourself" gives perspective on who and what you are. And it isn't that difficult. Doing a good hour's work or more will do it, providing service to others, laughing at yourself, going to a film, or doing anything else which absorbs your attention can serve the end of "getting out of yourself."

Be willing to take risks. Perhaps no one thing is more essential to growth than this. Earlier we discussed openness to challenge as one aspect of discipline. Being open to challenge is one kind of risk taking. Here, however, I am talking about a more general willingness to risk in diverse ways. Risk opening yourself up to a person who is not necessarily a close friend. Try a new way of doing things, a new system, a new route to work. Taking a new job is often a form of risk taking. Like everything else, risk taking can become an addiction, and the person who is constantly taking risks needs to consider what the meaning of that may be as well.

WHAT ABOUT THERAPY AND COUNSELING?

There will probably be times in either your emotional-spiritual development or during the progress of a relationship that it will be advisable to seek the help and support of a counselor or therapist. Identifying those times is usually not difficult if you are honest with yourself. If you experience uncontrollable fits of anger, deep sadness or depression, extreme frustration, lack of communication, physical abuse, persistent anxieties and fears, or repetitive patterns of manipulation, emotional harm, or unhelpful behavior, then you should consider therapy. At other times, despite the absence of such obvious indications, it may be just as helpful. So it is important to keep yourself open to the possibility that some kind of counseling or therapy might help.

In one or two sessions it is usually possible for the therapist to tell if someone can benefit from further therapy. There is probably seldom a time in people's lives where they can't learn something about themselves if they are open to it. If you try it at a time when you're not sure, the most you can lose is the cost of a couple of sessions. If in doubt, try it; it is rarely harmful (barring the choice of an unscrupulous therapist).

Usually much more difficult is the question of when to stop therapy. Most people want to stop before it is a good idea to do so. When you want to stop, be as sure as possible that the current material in your therapy isn't so threatening that it is easier not to confront it. Talk this point over specifically with your therapist. The decision to stop should be a "whole person" decision, made by your intellect, your emotions, and your spirit working together.

In this chapter I have outlined what I believe to be the traits or characteristics of the person whose emotional-spiritual health is good. There has been particular emphasis on spirituality, loving others, the importance of experiencing feelings, particularly anger and living for the present (day-tight compartments, doing it one day at a time). In addition to providing personal strength, these traits will also serve well in relationships with others, which is the topic of the next chapter.

RESOURCES CHAPTER 7

1. Emory, S. *Actualizations*. Garden City, New York: Doubleday Dolphin, 1978. A highly practical guide to personal growth and behavior in various applications.
2. Gibran, K. *The Prophet*. New York: Alfred Knopf, 1966. A classic volume of wisdom. Succint, universal, poetic.
3. Osler, W. *A Way of Life*. Baltimore, MD: The Remington-Putnam Book Company, 1932. Sir William's small but glittering gem on "day-tight compartments." An important basic strategy for mental health.
4. Peck. *The Road Less Traveled* (cited in Chapter 6).
5. Sehnert, K.W. *Stress/Unstress*. Minneapolis, MN: Augsburg, 1981. A compact and practical treatise on stress.

8

Healthy Relationships

DYNAMIC, growing relationships are a vital part of any normal person's life support system. They influence health and longevity, and are essential to the attainment of one's potential. Relationships need cultivation, fertilization, and care. Sometimes they need weeding. The rest of this section will help you learn the collective skills involved in doing these things — The Personal Health Competence of relationships. The focus is on close personal relationships with family and friends, but most of it applies to alliances with work colleagues as well.

THE BARSAL CONNECTION

The most remarkable intimacy I have known is that of my friends Barry and Sally. They are both in their 30's and have been together for about eight years. Their relationship is incredible simply because they work at it constantly, and they do good work. It has obviously paid off: they are close, open, trusting, and interdependent. They are beginning to look like each other.

The following aspects of their connectedness are exemplary. As individuals they each have that loving relationship with themselves that I spoke of before. Neither forgets that both of them are independent autonomous persons. Both accept their responsibility for the quality and value of the relationship between them. Their communication is clear and clean. Decisions which affect their life together are shared tirelessly. Sometimes this takes a lot of time, but it greatly enhances the quality of the rest of their hours together. When problems arise, they give top priority to resolving them. They are clear with one another regarding the goals, purposes, values, and expectations of their relationship. When they are not, they quickly spot it and get to work.

They support one another in myriad ways, which encompass practical matters, sensitivity to needs, affection, spiritual practices, and their work. For example, when Sally was a third-year student in medical school, she would come home and tell Barry what kinds of patients she had seen that day. He would humorously and lovingly lead her through a little catechism on two or three problems (he had been a physician for several years before Sal decided to go to medical school).

Last year they spent considerable time intricately planning a vacation to other parts of the country to visit relatives and friends. It was to take about two weeks and practically none of that time was to themselves. Two days before departure they picked up the tickets together and went out to lunch. Sally asked Barry how he was feeling about their plans and impending departure. "For some reason not very good," he replied. The conversation ended some hour and a half later. They cancelled their plans to visit everyone and took two weeks in their home state by themselves, mostly just relaxing.

Though very affectionate, they never appear cloying, overly demonstrative, or like they are playing to an audience. Hugging is commonplace in their household. They honor one another's feelings, even when what they feel is "bad energy" from the other person. Many times I have heard "in terms of what you just said I'm feeling some bad energy." Such a statement will be acknowledged, sometimes concurred with, sometimes not, and then the discussion goes on from there. In the earlier years of their relationship, while

trust was still developing, some discussions went on for a day or more until the nuances had been thoroughly worked out.

These words from *The Prophet* exemplify Sally and Barry's work and time together.

Love one another, but make not a bond of
   love:
Let it rather be a moving sea between the
   shores of your souls.
Fill each other's cup but drink not from one
   cup.
Give one another of your bread but eat not
   from the same loaf.
Sing and dance together and be joyous, but
   let each one of you be alone.
Even as the strings of a lute are alone though
   they quiver with the same music.
Give your hearts, but not into each other's
   keeping.
For only the hand of Life can contain your
   hearts.
And stand together, yet not too near together.
For the pillars of the temple stand apart,
And the oak tree and the cypress grow not
   in each other's shadow.

THE ESSENTIALS OF EMOTIONALLY HEALTHY RELATIONSHIPS

Certain elements or behaviors are common to successful alliances. What follows is an attempt to identify some guidelines which encompass them. Few relationships exhibit all of them. Some are easier to do than others. It may not be possible for partners to do some of these things together without help. People are so intricate and their old tapes and behavior patterns so well ingrained that using even the best guidelines effectively may be complicated and difficult. Unconscious themes and reaction patterns can interfere with, often block, the most sincere efforts to change. If this seems to be happening, it is a signal that you need help. On the other hand, there are those people for whom these common elements will be sufficient. They will be able to use them effectively and make profound progress.

Individual Traits

Chances for a successful alliance are greatly improved if each person comes to the affiliation with some or all of the following characteristics.

1. A loving relationship with self.
2. Firmly believing, like Barry and Sally, that you are directly responsible for the satisfaction/non-satisfaction, joy/non-joy, achievement/non-achievement of the alliance—that *nothing* that happens in a relationship is only one individual's responsibility.
3. Operating from your whole being: head (intellect), gut (feelings), and heart (spirit). This means as often and as consistently as possible operating from your center, that place that represents the integrated you, not just one aspect or another.

Collective Work

The rest of these guidelines are work to be done with your partner. When you use them, be sure that you decide together which ones you will work on. The most fundamental step in improving a relationship is to agree on what you're going to do.

1. Communicate well! Communication is a two-way street. All talking is not communicating, and talking is not the only way to communicate. Let's talk more about talking. Talk needs three qualities to be effective. First, it needs to be *clear*. Find the best words you can find to say what you want to say. If you say something and it doesn't sound like exactly what you meant to say, try again. It sometimes takes me three or four attempts to say what I want to say in a way that is clear to both me and my listener. If it sounds clear to you it is still important to "check it out" with the other person, particularly if it is an important point to have understood.

Second, talk should be *clean* (unclut-

tered). A lot of talk between people, especially that which is embedded in emotions or (particularly) that which directly expresses emotions, is not clean. It carries "old baggage" with it. Your partner does some relatively minor thing that irritates you. You complain much more vehemently than seems justified by the particular irritation. On that same day, work was tough. Your boss made you particularly angry during a discussion about vacations, but for valid reasons you decided not to express that anger at the time. It is still with you. The complaint you have made to your partner is carrying some of your anger at your boss along with it. That's not clean communication.

Third, talk should be *concise*. When you're talking about important things be brief. Sometimes, this is hard to do because you want to be complete. Or, one thing reminds you of something else that happened today. If your partner would rather hear more about that than stay on the initial matter, you've lost it.

In addition to talk, *listening* is an important part of communication. It is one of the hardest things to do well. Active listening involves really hearing what the other person has to say. It also requires genuinely experiencing and empathizing with the feelings imbedded in the words and the non-verbal behavior. Try sometime listening to someone for three minutes without interrupting them at all (tell them you're going to try this so that they won't be waiting for an answer). The first time you will use a lot of your attention and energy just to keep yourself quiet. Once you have mastered that, then start paying attention to what's being said. Hear both the message and the feelings that are included.

Finally, the skills of non-verbal communication are extremely important. If you do not get better and better each few months at sensing what's going on with your partner on the basis of facial expressions, moods, touches, hugs, and other forms of affection, then you're not improving your non-verbal skills.

2. Love and support one another. Earlier, love was defined as the commitment to support the growth of another person. In a relationship that extends over time, love is an on-going commitment to support the other's growth. You continuously find effective and helpful ways to support them, and by so doing love them in the deepest ways. One of the things that must be supported is individual autonomy ("And stand together, yet not too near together"). Many couples have difficulty in supporting one another's autonomy, i.e., they don't encourage and support whatever the other is doing as an individual. Barry supported Sally in every possible way during her journey through medical school. He was interested in knowing about what she was doing, helped her learn new material, and as far as possible arranged his free time to coincide with hers. In another couple by contrast, Jean subtly put down David's early attempts to become an entrepreneur in management consulting. At one point she called him "a loser."

Support can take many forms. Affection is one. Affirming and clarifying values is another. Financial and practical support can be provided. If your partner decides to make a change in his or her life, it is important to support that — if you ethically can, of course. Acknowledge progress and motion toward goals and finishing projects. When the person does something you don't like, be clear that it is the something, not them, that you don't like. Affirm their work. Validate their progress. Ask for their help with difficult tasks and ideas. Few things please me more in a relationship than being asked to help someone untangle their emotional turmoil or improve a term paper or listen to their newest ideas. People support me when they ask for my help.

Give support in being disciplined. The disciplines of self-responsibility, delayed gratification, openness to challenge, and honesty, which are so essential to personal emotional growth, must be encouraged. This is hard sometimes because it may conflict with something else you'd like to do. A simple example: Your friend has an exam at the end of the week. Your work schedule is light. You'd like to attend a concert and maybe a film during the week. Supporting the friend's effort to study before enjoying recreation (delaying gratification) is contrary to your wish to go to the concert and film with him.

3. Think context as well as content. The context of a relationship is elusive, all important, seldom explicit. In any relationship, people are aware of content. It is what we usually talk about. You are my boss. I am your employee. I do certain things for you: typing, running errands, leading projects, whatever I do for the job and whatever you do to be boss — that's the content. Both at work and at home, people live in and on the edge of the content of relationships. They discuss certain characteristics of one another or they argue about how this or that task got done and whether it got done right, or they agree about some of these things. "Why can't you get up on time to get my breakfast before I leave?" "I liked your report on the spono merger." "Do you think we should get a word processor in the back office?" All content.

What is context? It is the frame of reference within which people operate in a relationship. It includes goals (purposes), values, and expectations. Since (at least) two people are involved in a relationship the mutual clarification of context is critical to a healthy relationship, but this is seldom done. Perhaps working relationships are more often clear about context than personal ones. Often in a personal relationship the two parties are working with different contexts. If you asked either person a question about context (for example, the jointly shared goals of the relationship), they might be surprised to realize they hadn't discussed it. In a contemporary heterosexual partnership, for example, the man's goals are often sexual convenience, companionship at meals, good conversation. The woman, on the other hand, might have goals of emotional and physical security and entertaining. Now these two contexts are not necessarily mutually exclusive, but if there was not some communication and an attempt to move toward greater congruence, the relationship would most certainly founder.

Values are also an important part of context. If you take a new job as a salesman and value honesty, you may have a tough time relating with your boss (who also sells) and other salesmen who are willing to take liberties with the truth about your product in order to make a few more sales. Similarly for the last few years, I have worked in an educational center at a large health sciences teaching complex. I value changes in medical practice which nurture partnership between physicians and client (as contrasted with the expectation that people will simply do as the doctor tells them). These values do not have credibility or value in this medical center. They are not congruent with the tasks the center needs to do to serve the health science complex. This lack of common goals indicates that it is time to end the relationship and move on.

Similarly, expectations govern behavior in a powerful way, but are often not clear between the participants in a relationship. Women (less often men) in a relationship want and expect to be touched more than they are. But few of them say so directly. If you expect that your housemate will not read your mail, you may have to say so very clearly. If you're expecting to use the car this weekend instead of leaving it up for grabs by your husband and all of the teenagers, it will help immensely if you say so clearly and often enough that it is not forgotten. If you expect to get half a morning off every three weeks to go to your physician, you had better discuss it with your supervisor.

Many people who enter relationships are emotionally-spiritually bankrupt and sick enough that they are not even aware of their part in defining context. They are operating from needs that they either do not acknowledge or have not perceived. In such relationships the most damaging manipulation probably occurs. Someone who explicity manipulates at least has some conscious direction to his gyrations and, if confronted, may acknowledge what he wants.

SOME MAJOR STUMBLING BLOCKS IN RELATIONSHIPS

Although the differences between true intimacy and manipulative dependency without intimacy are significant, the two are often subjectively confused by lovers or partners. Sex and sexuality are another major problem in many relationships. Less tenacious, very common, and often unrecognized stumbling blocks are the tendency for putting the other person down and for trying to change them.

Some Reflections on Intimacy and Dependency

Intimacy might be regarded as the ultimate goal of many friendships, marriages, and other partnering arrangements. Some alliances do progress to genuine intimacy: the partners share closeness, they are open and candid with one another, they have mutual trust, and they are interdependent. Not all of these charac-

88 THE PATHWAY OF EMOTIONAL-SPIRITUAL HEALTH

teristics will be equally strong, but to some degree they will all be present if a relationship is intimate.

Durability of a relationship alone is *not* evidence for intimacy. Many couples who have been together for a decade or more are far from intimate. For many people true intimacy is frightening and its prospect interferes with the progress of a relationship. The possibility of openness and healthy interdependence may be too threatening or sufficient trust impossible to attain.

Students of relationships and intimacy believe that the nature of an infant's relationship with its primary caretaker, usually the mother, determines the capacity of that individual for later intimacy. They say that if true intimacy was not present in a person's relationship with their caretaker(s), it cannot be attained later, unless some kind of significant growth experience (like therapy) intervenes. I agree with this. I do not know of a rich and lasting intimate relationship in which both partners have not had either an extraordinarily good relationship with their mother or some kind of psychotherapeutic experience.

Because dependency needs are natural and universal, but often the seat or target of manipulative behaviors, pathological dependency is frequently a disruptive force in relationships. All of us depend on others. When we are small, our needs include being fed and cleaned, affection, love, and protection. In later life, we depend on others for approval, support, affection, attention, help in growing, and satisfaction of other needs.

When dependency needs are so powerful as to govern a person's behavior or when they are denied entirely, they can disrupt relationships. Pathological dependency exists when a person's need to depend on others reaches a level where they can do little if anything by themselves. This sometimes makes it impossible for the supporter(s) to function normally.

Overly dependent people behave in some (or all) ways like children. They require constant attention, the presence of another person, constant praise, or other kinds of gratification. They become skilled manipulators to attain those goals. This is a difficult situation for everyone involved, and the dependent person requires therapy.

As difficult, but usually more subtle, is the person who denies normal or increased need for dependency. Many people with normal dependency needs do not admit or "own" them (particularly adolescent and adult males). In much of our culture, it is considered "sissy" or "weak" to be dependent or acknowledge dependency. So a lot of men and some women deny their dependency needs. The danger of denial is that the dependency needs are expressed in some unclear or confusing way. It may be as a tendency to overcontrol, as extreme anxiety when the partner is away from home, or in any number of other ways.

The following passage emphasizes these points:

Altruistic loving, or the self-giving type of caring, is not a selfish process. Yet some people 'love' selfishly, and their emotionally driven sense of possessiveness and expectations centers on 'need.' They *need* their partner's attention, presence, and performance to satisfy their own desires. Varah states that " 'love' seeks to give what the other wants and to take what the other person wants to give. *Need* seeks to get what it wants and to give only what it chooses to give . . ."

An extreme degree of need may be harmful, but all people have needs, and (partners) rightfully expect to have them met. To the extent that need expectations are mutually fulfilled, the individuals benefit and the (partnership) is strengthened; unfulfilled needs create resentment and displeasure, and the relationship deteriorates.[1]

1. Marital Problems (a booklet), Medical Datamation, Bellevue, Ohio, 1976 (no author given). The author is grateful to the Editorial Staff of Medical Datamation, Bellevue, Ohio, for permission to quote this passage from the pamphlet entitled "Marital Problems," 1976.

On Changing Others

The desire to change others probably causes more difficulty in relationships than any other thing. Judging others, comparing yourself to others (or others to others), and taking people's inventories are all "natural" activities. We all do them well. The catch is that they usually precede me trying to change you. My ego is what really wants to change you. It puffs me up if I "suggest" a change, and you change (or appear to change).

Regardless of why people want to change each other, the tools are control, force, and manipulation. Manipulation is often preferred because it's not so obvious. If I don't "control" you or "force" you, I'm still a "good guy." So I'll manipulate (a sophisticated form of control) you instead. So it gets to be a game. The fact is that no one will change until they are ready.

Think of a plant. You can't *make* a plant grow or flower. You can provide water, soil, light, and nutrients, or create adverse conditions by withholding these essentials. You can encourage the plant's growth or kill it. But you can't *make* it grow or flower differently than it's innate knowledge and process do. People are the same. You can facilitate their self-selected change or growth. You may inform them of choices they didn't know they had, but if you *force* change, you will stunt them.

We often want to change people for loving reasons, particularly when they are doing something clearly bad for themselves. Smoking is an excellent example. You want your partner, let's say, to stop "for their own good." But it's tricky because often you also want them to stop because it bothers you—the smoke, their coughing, and the taste of their breath. I heard of a woman who smoked in the closet (actually!) for five years, so her husband, who wanted her to stop, wouldn't know she was still smoking. She used deodorants and air fresheners, and had her clothes cleaned frequently. She finally gave up and really stopped—it was all too much trouble. But for 5 years she lived that complicated lie because her husband wanted her to change, and she wanted him to think that she had.

Emotional-spiritual issues can be even trickier. If someone treats their kids badly, any attempt to get them to change runs the risk of being labeled as "butting in on something that isn't your business," or it is felt as a direct assault on their character.

This does not mean that you shouldn't inform people. If someone isn't aware that smoking is bad for them or that they continually put their kids down, then, if you love them, you will need to make it clear. But not with the expectation that they will change. That's the difference. The responsibility for informing them is one thing. It is a way in which you can be "present" or helpful. The responsibility for actually making the change is the other person's. It helps me not to try to change you, if I can remember that.

If a single rule were selected to govern all relationships, it might well be "accept people as they are; don't try to change them." But how do you stop wanting someone to be different? How can you support another's growth without wanting them to change? How do I stop taking responsibility for your life as well as my own?

If I want or need someone to change, I try to be honest about it and at the same time say that I'm going to try to "let go" of the need. Then I clearly separate my love and valuing of him or her as a person from how I feel about the thing he or she is doing. "Mike, I love you, but I sure don't like it when you smoke so much pot." This takes away the threat that the continued behavior may cause the loss of my love. Then they can enlist my assistance in making the change. At the least, it has eliminated a lot of ambivalence and guilt.

It also helps to remember that I'm not perfect. When I'm being honest with myself that's not hard to do. Once I remember that I'm not perfect, then somehow our differences don't seem nearly as important. But the thing that works best for me is to pray — to ask God for the grace not to try to change you, but only to be present and to change myself if that's what is really needed. And then what happens? I either lose the need to change you or decide to change myself. Or I choose not to stick around — that's my choice too.

A person has to change themselves. We can't change each other. In that spirit just take from here what you want, contact my center, acknowledge my words, honor my destination and move on. My investment is not in whether you change. Were you present?

Sex and Sexuality

Sex is a central issue for most of us. Complicated! It probably causes more problems in emotional maturation and development than anything else. A lot of this trouble is due to our internal conflicts about it and more is related to conflicts (spoken and unspoken, perceived and unperceived) we have with our partners over it. Perhaps it is no accident that the word *sex* is derived from a Latin-Middle English root, "akin to secus which is a derivative of 'secare', to cut, divide."

The amount of ego most men (and some women) have invested in sexual performance is large. We are preoccupied with "scoring," performance, failure, setting it up, and "getting it off." We think much less in terms of creativity, beauty, and commitment when sex is concerned. For many people, sex has become objectified and trivialized — it is a commodity. Since the cornerstone of Personal Health Competence and wellness

are integration, creativity, change, and wholeness, it seems as though sex, as a basic and potentially beautiful part of our existence, should be part of our wholeness too, not outside it.

George Leonard's book, *The End of Sex*,[1] states strong views and presents them well. Leonard welcomed the sexual revolution. Among other things, "it freed us after years of repression to discuss sexual matters, to live together openly without marriage, and to enjoy our erotic utopia . . . Not quite."[2] He goes on to describe the backlash — from the Moral Right and its allies in government. In addition, he points out, there has been "sleaziness" and exploitation. Biology has now also dampened utopian hopes for free love with an epidemic of genital herpes and, more recently, the lethal Acquired Immune Deficiency Syndrome (AIDS). But for Leonard, these are not the reasons the revolution will fail. He sees the problem as the structure of the reform movement itself. "Victorian proscription has been replaced by subtle but pervasive prescription." That is, the terrifying Victorian injunctions against masturbation have given way to dogma that it is good therapy, good self-relaxation, good political statement, "*duty*." Assumptions, such as pleasure and satisfaction are the chief aims of sexual activity, have become ideology, then dogma. "In the minds and practices of the reformers, sex has long been separated from love"; it has also been divorced from creation and disconnected from procreation (the latter is mentioned in very few books on sex), and other social and ethical considerations. So come to believe that our erotic behavior actually has little to do with anything else we believe, feel, or do — it is trivial, and impersonal.

Sex can be an activity of great love,

1. George Leonard, *The End of Sex* (Los Angeles: J.P. Tarcher, 1983).
2. Ibid, p.9.

sensitivity, creativity, and compassion, an integrative act. Or, it can be automatic, manipulative, controlling, objectified, and trivialized. It can be angry, hateful, and physically destructive, or it can be healing.

For many, sex has become an isolated experience not integrated with commitment, apart from love. It's not often or ever the creative (not procreative) experience that it can be. It is a commodity that we bargain for rather than a central creative force in our lives. In contrast, since the running boom began, many people have continued to run because it is an integrating experience for them. They think, create, and plan while they are running. It is an experience of wholeness, not just one of sweat.

One difficult thing about sex is that it can be *so* powerful. At orgasm, as Peck says, our ego barriers fall away. Our defenses and protection dissolve in that moment. We merge with time and space. The moment has been aptly called La Petite Mort. Therefore, while exciting and intensely beautiful, it can be felt or anticipated at some level as an experience of the most frightening kind.

It is also developmentally charged. We experience it as pleasant or exciting: we want it, and our peers encourage us to participate. At the same time, we're frightened by family and cultural strictures. Most of us have been conditioned by our parents to be secretive about it or told (explicitly or implicitly) that it's bad or we're too young. We become timid, shy, withdrawn, and incomplete. Thus, the sheer power and vulnerability of the experience and the culturally induced inhibitions about it may combine to have the vulnerable and frightening aspects seem like punishment. This can add to the confusion.

I was eight before either parent ever mentioned sex to me. My mother had remarried when I was five and it was three more years before my sister arrived. That seemed like a long time. I thought the reason I didn't get a sibling was because "making" one was so unpleasant and painful. Somewhere I had learned that the father had to put his penis "inside" the mother and the thought of that happening with my parents was chilling to me.

One night I asked my mother why I had not been circumcised. She said, "So that intercourse will be more exciting for you." I was flabbergasted. This was totally opposed to my notion of what must be going on. When I said so, she seemed surprised and assured me that intercourse was wonderful.

After that episode, the blackout resumed despite the fact that mother now knew how ignorant I was. I learned a little from my friends and a little here and there from books. The Boy Scout Manual had a piece on masturbation titled "Conservation." It was archaic, right out of a Victorian censure essay. It was so bad that even I, impressionable as I was, didn't quite believe it could all be true. But I believed enough of it that it increased my guilt for at least a decade.

So, I masturbated surreptitiously for years with enormous amounts of guilt, terrified that I would be discovered. I sent for postcards of naked women and occasionally talked about sex with my friends. I neither read nor was told anything that was positively helpful in any way. I was convinced for years that I should "save" myself for marriage. Though not necessarily an unhelpful idea (I now believe), it came then from fear. By the time I was in medical school that notion had changed, but then I was unable to have more than a few minutes of erotic petting without premature ejaculation. It was not until many months after marriage that I was more "normal."

As the years went by I became what might be called an adult soldier in the sexual revolution. I had affairs, always with great guilt, never recognizing my deep underlying problems with intimacy and commitment. After divorce, my attitudes toward sex were schizophrenic. At times I would trivialize and objectify it. When in a seemingly solid relationship, I would feel, by contrast, that sex was an integral part of that relationship and my life, that it could not be separated as a commodity to partake of at any whim, and that monogamy made sense.

In the last three years, I have worked hard on my emotional-spiritual blocks with respect to commitment, intimacy, and partnering. There has been substantial success. I feel ready to make a lasting commitment in a partnering relationship. My fear of intimacy, although rearing its stubborn head at times, is basically resolved. What went before is instructive, but largely in the sense of how it might have been different.

Because of my own unfavorable experiences, I resolved that my own children would fare better with respect to their education and understanding about sex. I think they did, but only because of the more freely available information, not because of help I provided. If I could have the chance again, here are the things I would tell them.

1. The sexual experience is a wonderful, important, and normal *part of life.* It can be a rich part of loving someone, in the sense I have used that phrase before.
2. Sexual activity is richest as an integrated life experience. While "casual" sex may not be unhelpful per se, it often reflects fractionation of one's life and an attitude of objectification, which if habitual may not encourage normal development.
3. It is requisite to a healthy sex life that everyone freely choose when they begin, under what circumstances, and

with what sex. An aware "whole person" decision to embrace the homosexual experience deserves the same celebration as one to be heterosexual. There is no one way of sexual being that is best for everyone — or even for the same person at different times in his or her life.

4. The responsibility and respect that sex entails towards the partner should be emphasized and lived. You do not lead another person to one of the most vulnerable places in life without abundant care, attention, and responsibility. Cajoling and manipulation are not healthy, responsible behaviors. The other person's wishes and preferences should be respected. The decision to have or not have sex needs to be a mutual one. If either person says "no," that should be honored.
5. Masturbation is a normal dimension of a healthy and loving relationship with yourself. It is a way of loving and caring for yourself and helps you to learn about your body's sexual responses. It lets you enjoy sex when you are not part of a relationship that is sexual, but can be part of a continuing relationship with yourself when you are also part of an active relationship with another. As with all aspects of sex, masturbation should be a personal choice. A choice of abstention, like a choice of celibacy, is to be honored and respected.
6. There is no question that wider and more effective dissemination of information will be very helpful in the overall picture. But information alone is not *nearly* enough, even if it is of the best kind and most competently delivered. Education is more than that. Those purporting to provide "sex education" need to remember that sensitive exploration of the gut and the heart as well as the mind is essential. Feelings need to be recognized,

discussed, and honored. Values must be probed and clarified. One's faith must be clear.

In the definitive reckoning, perhaps we will comprehend more clearly that sex above all else is a whole person activity that involves complex physiologic and neurologic changes, deep moral conditioning, and (for most of us) religious or spiritual concepts that are soundly based. For any given individual, this complexity must be recognized, indeed celebrated. We need, as Leonard says, something beyond the sexual revolution which can begin with a new way of perceiving and conceptualizing the erotic realm, "not another turn of the wheel of repression and liberation."

Putting People Down

A common way of relating to others is the put-down. Many adults are practiced and skillful at putting people down. And children learn fast. Putting someone down is a manifestation of the anger-fear energy and an active process of non-valuing. It is targeted at people in all stages of life. Instead of celebrating the value and beauty in one another, we put each other down.

Unless your parents were unusual, they probably put you down often. If they were subtle about it, you may not remember. A common one is, "You're not old enough to do that." How many times are children not old enough to do how many different things? Stay up late with the adults; ride a bicycle; go to the store alone. "You wouldn't understand" is another. Argghh. "What do you mean I wouldn't understand; how do you *know* I wouldn't understand? Try me! If you won't even try me, you must not value my abilities or even think I *might* be able to do it."

And here's one I've watched happen to others. At the same time in life they're

being told "you're not old enough" or "you wouldn't understand," they also hear "you need to grow up." "John, why don't you grow up   you act so immature." Yeah, right! John's not old enough to travel alone because you won't give him that responsibility, but he needs to grow up because he's acting immature. Catch 22!

A lot of put-downs are intellectual. They may be quite direct ("You don't know what you're talking about.") or conveyed through an irritated or condescending tone of voice. Just dominating the conversation can put people down. However it happens, the effect is one of discounting your opinion or ideas.

Even though each individual put-down seems relatively insignificant, the net effect day after day is one huge self-fulfilling prophecy. It is terrible for self-esteem. After a time, the child feels and acts like a loser. It is a great leveling process. Instead of being helped toward deeper and richer places in life, the person is put down.

A very common form of put-down is teasing. Some families communicate mainly through teasing. This is damaging. Sure, there is a place for teasing. Here and there, if it's done in a loving way, it can be fun and helpful. But when it carries misplaced anger, fear, or jealousy, it's another form of put-down. "Oh, Waysie's got shorts on again today," or "You couldn't make the team with an elephant glove." I grew to hate teasing so much that I couldn't recognize loving humor. Any teasing represented an attack. Several years ago I met Larry who taught me it didn't have to be that way, but it sure took a while to learn.

A dangerous thing about teasing is that it can become a context for life. If all communication takes place in the context of teasing, it's hard to attach degrees of importance to things. It's all a big joke.

Putting someone down is done with

behavior as well as words. If you don't listen attentively when your teenager is trying to talk to you about his new girlfriend, a course at school, or plans for vacation, then that clearly puts him down. You're devaluing his concern, involvement, or investment. By devaluing his concerns, you devalue your relationship with him. You've got to be there.

A more subtle form of put-down is to guide a child or adult too closely through something new. The kids never get a chance to try out their own ideas about how it should be done. If you're a parent or "friend" who doesn't let people try new things in their way, you are putting them down. They may end up plastic and moldable and demure — or rebellious. It's no wonder children rebel. They want to get away from situations in which they are controlled and not valued. They are told when and where and for how long they can do what, and their own ideas and abilities are not appreciated or are overtly put down. And the saddest part of all is that whatever you do to your children they'll probably do to theirs. Then, of course, you can criticize them for doing the same things you always did to them. Fun!

Relationships are as basic to our emotional-spiritual health as food is to our bodies. They are a source of great love and enrichment, and they cause frustration, conflict, and pain. Certain guidelines have been presented which, if followed, will increase the love and enrichment of relationships and substantially reduce the pain and problems. Issues on which relationships can founder are intimacy and dependency, sex and sexuality, put-downs and changing others. Some of the intricacies surrounding these stumbling blocks have been clarified and caution signals identified. Building healthy relationships is difficult but rewarding work that never ends.

The next chapter talks about specialized relationships with systems and individuals (advocates) who may support you in your quest for Personal Health Competence.

RESOURCES CHAPTER 8

1. Bell, R. *Changing Bodies, Changing Lives.* New York: Random House, 1980.
2. Gibran. *The Prophet* (cited in Chapter 7).
3. Klimek, D., Ph.D. *Beneath Mate Selection and Marriage: The Unconscious Motives in Human Pairing.* New York: Van Nostrand-Reinhold, Co., 1979. An illuminating and detailed analysis of what brings couples together and moves them apart. Not always easy reading.
4. Leonard, G. *The End of Sex.* Los Angeles: J.P. Tarcher (Houghton Mifflin), 1983. This book is quoted above. It is a useful, fresh and penetrating look at the sexual revolution and what can lie beyond — asking how we can again make sex an integral part of our lives rather than a stylized, objectified activity.

9

Advocacy and People-Support Systems

YOUR personal support system consists of people resources and non-people resources. This chapter is about people-support systems. Learning to use and maximally benefit from the support of others is a vital part of being health competent.

Two basic kinds of people support are helpful for increasing health and coping with illness: individuals and groups. An advocate is a special kind of supporting individual, and networks are a special kind of group. Some people are more comfortable with an individual as the mainstay of their support system; others prefer groups. However, I believe many people tend to develop fixed patterns of interaction when they rely too heavily on only one individual. This can impede growth. I recommend an overall support system which includes two or three important individuals, one high-priority group, and as many other groups and networks as you need.

While it is obvious that the support of others is emotionally and spiritually strengthening, many of us, paradoxically, have difficulty accepting such support. This phenomenon is related to the strong cultural value attached to "doing it alone."

ON DOING IT ALONE

For most of my life I have been a "loner." As a boy I spent a lot of time alone. This pattern continued for many years. It was particularly evident when I needed help or comfort as a result of emotional upset, loss, frustration, or confusion. To endure alone was the "strong way, the good way, the best way." Only it wasn't.

Twice during my life, I have suffered prolonged and deep depression. The first time I was too fearful to seek help and, as a consequence, suffered longer than I needed to. The second time I was obsessed with suicidal thoughts until I became scared enough to go to a psychiatrist. With his support and skill, I eventually overcame my fears and desolation.

Vestiges of the tendency to isolate are still with me. Certain crises click on the same old tape: "get away, don't speak to anyone, fix it yourself." I must fight these inclinations. Now most clearly, *I have a choice*. I can identify my tendency to isolate or the fact that I am isolating, and at least choose whether to continue or not.

This tendency to "do it alone" is quite common, particularly in men. Men "don't cry" or express "soft" emotions, and they don't ask for help. Women, as a rule, cry more openly and more easily ask for support from friends or relatives, although not always clearly.

Isolating is closely related to doing it alone. Isolating is a process whereby an individual withdraws and experiences neither self nor the outside world. It is a way of being stuck in one's relationship with self and with others. Solitude, on the other hand, is a health-giving experience, freely chosen, which serves the purpose of stimulating self-awareness and personal growth that can sometimes not be stimulated in any other way. Solitude facilitates the experience of one's self thereby permitting self-growth, which, in turn, enriches subsequent experiences with the world.

WHY SEEK HELP FROM OTHERS

Love and interdependence are powerful modes of human expression. This is why societies and families and other natural groupings occur. The idea that being dependent on someone is weak doesn't make sense. We all have needs for attachment. Everyone needs to depend on others, to have others in their lives for support, friendship, comfort, and physical affection. The feeling of support by other people perhaps does more than any other thing to assuage and diminish, indeed completely dissolve, the fear of being alone.

When one is ill, as opposed to being engaged in health activities, these needs are often greater. If you are in a coma, unable to talk because of a stroke, or so preoccupied with pain that you can't think about anything else, then the need for an advocate (an ally who has your specific interests at heart with the specific talents to support them) is obvious. You need someone who thinks like you and who knows you pretty well to speak up for you and to help make decisions about what is going to happen to you. You need a representative in the truest sense of the word. In such a dependent situation, an advocate can fulfill your dependency needs. Your advocate should be someone you trust. It is usually more satisfactory and safer to let a trusted advocate fill your needs than a stranger.

In addition to situations of physical handicap or helplessness, one may also be psychologically helpless or dysfunctional. Fear, anxiety, pain, anger, and loneliness can all make you feel helpless. In addition, strong emotions may make you non-assertive or verbally aggressive. Your medical care provider may then react instead of responding helpfully. In either case, your position will be weakened and the chance your best interests will be secured becomes minimized. Under such circumstances an advocate can be extremely helpful.

People-support systems can also provide encouragement and companionship. Both recovery from illness and the adoption of a new health-giving activity require energy and faith. The encouragement of others or another during the ordeal of illness, particularly during hospitalization, is invaluable. The encouragement that can be provided by a companion (either another neophyte or one who has attained some competence) during the acquisition of a new health habit or a change in habits is similarly important. I have seen many people who had tried repeatedly, over long periods of time, to make changes alone and failed, later to succeed in the company of a partner or a group who were making the same change.

Finally, we know that physical touching is essential to normal life development. Infants who are not touched quickly become ill and die. People who have physical companionship over long continuous periods live longer and stay healthier. The touching and care of the mind and the spirit must be equally important if not more so. Support systems can, with their other more tangible functions, provide such touching and care of the mind and spirit. In my view, this is ultimately their most important function.

CHARACTERISTICS OF EFFECTIVE SUPPORT SYSTEMS

The following list of "support group functions" is not all inclusive. Nor is a person or group not doing its job if it doesn't do all of these things. The list is focused on support groups for health activities but applies to support groups in general. It will help you think about your own support network in terms of what you would like it to be doing, compare that with what you think it is doing, and think about how you might make up the important deficits if that can be done. Don't forget to add additional purposes of your own if you wish to.

Support System Functions

1. Provide unqualified personal regard. This means valuing each individual as a precious, important person, as an equal who has something to offer (even though in the beginning that may be relatively minimal) as well as needs to be met.

2. Accept each individual in a non-judgmental and non-evaluative way (it is particularly important that feelings not be judged; they cannot be changed anyway). This does not mean that persons may not have to be told or advised that a certain behavior or plan is not helpful, not in their best interests, or that there are more effective ways of doing certain things. However, with respect to a person's choices and behaviors, judgments should be kept to a minimum. They should not be moralistic, but made in terms of how helpful or non-helpful the behavior is to the individual being "judged."

3. Give empathy without pity. This involves "walking in another person's shoes" and trying to feel what they are feeling. It requires living their experience and helping from that place rather than "feeling sorry for them."

4. Be enthusiastic about whatever a person is doing, as insignificant as the activity may seem, as long as it is not unhelpful to them.

5. Provide physical comfort and affection. There are situations where this is inappropriate, but they are few (contrary to what it seems when watching people's behavior). This can include touching, embracing, or holding someone's hand.

6. Set limits, and be clear about what they are. Almost all support groups need limits on behavior, but often they don't need very many.

7. Help process feelings, disappointments, and frustrations over life events. Often this involves little more than listening attentively and giving your presence to an individual. It may also include clarifying, summarizing, and making suggestions for further investigation or choices in behavior.

8. Provide specific information and advice about the particular illness or problem for which the group exists. For example, if the group is a diabetes group, then a newcomer would be educated by the group regarding the disease itself and its management.
9. Give encouragement (usually as a later task) to all of its members to get out of themselves — to support others, to work effectively, to play hard.

All of these functions cannot be performed by single individuals and rarely by one group. We learn through mistakes and "failures"; everyone must hear how to do it and then try to do it, and no one will be perfect about anything. In a well functioning group, someone will be available for the kind of help you need at any given time, when you need it; someone who has had a similar problem or stuck place will tell you how they managed.

Support Networks

Support networks consist of one or more people who support you in terms of a specific work or health function. They may never meet, or if they do, it will be infrequently as a whole group. They function primarily through the mail, by telephone, or by meetings of two or more individuals who then communicate with others in the network. For example, I have a network of people whom I contact and work with in relation to the issues of making medicine more caring, another that helps me learn more about brain dominance, and a third in health competence and health promotion (the realm of this book). Very few people are in more than one of the three networks. I seldom have interactions with these people except in relationship to those issues.

Support and Therapy Groups

Unlike networks, most groups meet regularly. They may be the same people each time (in the case of small local organizations) or the "membership" of any one group may be variable and constantly fluid (which is the case with many disease-focused support groups). Groups may have a specific purpose or a broader function. Many which ostensibly focus on one problem actually serve a broader function. Alcoholics Anonymous, for example, is focused on the specific task of helping people stay sober but serves the much broader function of helping people live spiritually healthy lives.

Groups provide a safe forum for processing your own problems, fears, experiences, hopes, and joy about certain aspects of your life. Group therapy is a kind of whole-life support group. People grow by having their own needs met and by working through problems. But they also grow by getting out of themselves and by helping others.

Support from Individuals

All of us have friends and family members who support us. They contribute to our health by providing psychological support and companionship or encouragement in the pursuit of healthy habits. They may also help us in specific ways when we are ill.

Health (or illness) advocates are people we enlist to support us specifically in health activities or during illness. They may or may not be drawn from among friends and family members. They can, for example, provide encouragement and companionship for exercise or eating well. They are available to support your interactions with medical care providers, including speaking and acting on your behalf when necessary.

An advocacy is a working alliance built around the goal of personal health and health competence. (You may have bought a used car and in the process had a trusted mechanic or friend check it out and advise you; this is an example of advocacy.) A counselor or psychotherapist is a special kind of advocate who provides some of the functions mentioned earlier in this chapter, but focuses on your emotional health, helping you cope more effectively, dissipate anxiety and fear, and move from a place of anger and hostility to one of love and peace — particularly with yourself.

The rest of this chapter talks about advocates who are not professional health providers. The use of counselors and psychotherapists is discussed at the end of Chapter 7 (Individual Emotional-Spiritual Health).

SELECTING AND USING AN ADVOCATE

An advocate must be someone you trust. Those closest to us may not always be the best choice, though often they are. They cannot always be uninvolved enough to press for the decisions we want.

Clem is my very close friend, a physician, and my own age. He has all my passion for personal health competence. Two years ago he had coronary artery by-pass surgery, and I served as his advocate. One day after surgery he was drugged, in pain, and miserable. Seeing him in this way, I was not entirely sure that my attachment to him wouldn't encourage me to grasp at therapeutic straws if he worsened, rather than press for the decisions I knew he would favor.

It is important to choose an advocate with the understanding that either party can fire the other at any time. You should choose someone who can and will commit the time that it takes to be a good advocate. The expectations you have of your advocate must be clarified. If they are not, you will probably be disappointed, and your advocate will be confused and feel badly for having failed to live up to your expectations. Try to predict problems and events and be prepared to deal with them. Meet regularly

even if there are not new changes in the situation. A good advocate will perform some or all of the following functions:

1. Help you clarify your expectations and philosophy about medical care; part of this task is to recite back your expectations and philosophy and help you evaluate it.
2. Participate with you in new healthy activities (if you are both beginners you can support one another).
3. Plan visits to your physician or other health care provider and accompany you on these visits whenever necessary (sometimes this is regularly).
4. Help you evaluate your progress in health-giving activities or physician interactions.
5. When you are faced with hospitalization, discuss carefully with you your reasons for going there, expectations of the experience and providers, your medical problem and what you both know about it, procedures to be performed, and your philosophy about extreme measures.

A good advocate will serve as an extension of you and as an interpreter for you. During medical care, especially in the hospital, he or she will not allow things to happen that you oppose. The guidelines just given will help you get what you want and achieve an effective working relationship.

If you are being hospitalized under the care of a specialist, your family physician may be able to serve as your advocate. This can be a very satisfactory situation, but often a family physician is too busy.

Mutual advocacy is suggested for those of you who really have trouble with the whole idea of being supported. In mutual advocacy there is equality. In certain situations you will be the support and advocate and in others your partner will be, creating a healthy state of interdependence. When the need arises in either direction for support, it is available. Partners or spouses can be mutual advocates. Mutual advocacy still takes preparation: you will need to clarify objectives, predict problems, and schedule meetings. There are always certain points which may never have been discussed and others which need reinforcement.

PROBLEMS ENCOUNTERED IN SUPPORT SYSTEMS

Everyone has dependency needs — needs for comfort, affection, love, and attention. Their healthy fulfillment is part of everyday living. A well person clearly appreciates such needs and makes choices about how to respond to them. However, some people ignore these dependency needs by not admitting them to awareness or denying their importance. They "do it alone" when they could benefit from support. They may be in a support system but unable to use it. (See Chapter 8 on Relationships.)

Other people have an exaggerated and abnormal expression of dependency needs. We say they are "needy." Neediness occurs when a certain need becomes a person's central focus and its fulfillment an obsession or preoccupation. *Choices* are not made by people under such circumstances — they only react to their neediness. This can be extremely uncomfortable, frustrating, and aggravating for the supporting person or system. They, in turn, may react with irritation, outright anger, or manipulation, and aggravate the problem. They do not reach out when they themselves could benefit from support, and they may become reluctant to be a support person in more normal situations.

An abnormally needy person can be helped by a group. The best strategy is for one individual to provide special attention (sponsorship) and be the lead person, supplemented with help from others so that no one individual becomes too angry or turned off by the excessive dependence of the needy one. A group can help the needy one understand what situations create his neediness; the needy one can then begin to learn to make other choices when those situations arise.

Unfortunately, all support systems are not altruistic. Groups can become self-aggrandizing and subordinate, exploit, or brainwash their supporters. Cults are a good example of how support groups can be aggrandizing. They lure unsuspecting, needy individuals into their sphere of influence, indoctrinate them, and then exploit them by having them work for nothing or recruit other newcomers. Individual support people probably err most often by controlling and dominating rather than by facilitating growth and healing. Some do this unconsciously to fulfill their own needs to be important to someone or to control others.

It is not always easy to identify support people or systems that are defective in these ways. Elements of secrecy, dogma, proselytization (if you say no, they don't give up), and lack of a track record are all clues that should alert you to be cautious with groups or organizations. Apparent neediness, excessively controlling activity and attitude, dogmatism, poor listening ability, unwillingness to discuss one's own shortcomings are all characteristics that suggest personal inadequacy in the case of would-be individual supporters.

Some people join or solicit the help of a support group, only to run after getting their "hit." One of the long-term benefits of group support is the confidence, grace, and self-knowledge that derives from helping others with the same or similar problems. Consider carefully whether your responsibility to the group has been fulfilled before you leave.

Willingness to accept the help and support of others is an essential ingredient in health-giving activities, particularly those of emotional-spiritual health. The tendency to isolate and do it alone is a strong one in our society, especially among males.

For some health activities and illnesses, an individual supporter or advocate probably works best. In other situations, groups seem to do a better job. Everyone has to learn what is best for himself or herself.

RESOURCES CHAPTER 9

Borman, L. (Ed.) *Helping People to Help Themselves: Self-Help and Prevention.* New York: The Haworth Press, 1982.

Lieberman, M.A. and Borman, L.D. *Self-Help Groups for Coping with Crisis.* San Francisco, CA: Jossey-Bass, 1979.

The Self-Help Group Consortium (Helping People Help Themselves) (see General Resources, Organizations).

Part ***IV***

THE PATHWAY OF EATING, MOVING, AND HABITS

THE MASTERY OF unhealthy habits, sound body structure, physical conditioning, good nutrition, and weight management are the subjects of Part IV. Except for sound body structure, they are the aspects of health and health promotion that we hear most about these days.

Unhealthy habits are just that. They lead to premature disease, disability, and death. More importantly, they take time, sap energy, and often contribute to depression. Many are outright addictions, and the rest have characteristics of addictions. Basically, the chapter on unhealthy habits is a treatise on how to change. The successful incorporation of most other health competencies into your life-style will involve change, and the process is outlined in this section.

Sound body structure is a combination of good body alignment and flexibility-muscle balance. These attributes protect against vast numbers of aches and pains, avoid many injuries, and significantly prolong good function in both work and play. Sound structure boosts the psyche as well. Sound structure is, however, only part of "being in shape." Aerobic conditioning and good muscle tone developed through exercise and movement are the other essential components of true physical fitness.

Good healthy food provides the energy we need in accordance with good nutritional principles, safety, and lasting health. Weight management, important for several health reasons, is perhaps most important to more people because of the cultural pressure to be slim and trim. There is confusion today over what is and what is not healthy regarding fat. The chapter on weight management is primarily based on the assumption that too much fat is not healthy, but it also recognizes the need to seriously examine certain important challenges to that basic assumption.

103

It would be misleading to think of this pathway as the "body" section in any sharp contrast to the "mind-spirit" section which has just proceeded it. The previous part did concentrate on the spiritual and feeling part of our being and existence, and this part does focus on more physical ones. But the activities and skills described here provide mental stimulation, relaxation, and freedom from anxiety for the mind and spirit. Contrary to a lot of current cultural fitness dogma, the foundation of health and wellness is in the synergy of mind and body, not simply in the muscles.

10

Changing Unhealthy Habits

AS emphasized in Chapter 2 (Taking Your Inventory of Health, Well-being, and Problems), future health problems are determined by age, sex, race, the family medical history, and personal habits or behaviors. In terms of staying healthy and improving well-being, a person has no control over any of these except personal habits and behaviors. In that arena, however, we can profoundly influence our own health and well-being. Healthy behaviors are obviously an important category of health competence, but changing unhealthy behaviors is not an easy task. This chapter takes a look at why that is and offers suggestions to improve your chances for successful change. Changing and adjusting are truly skills of Personal Health Competence.

In some people unhealthy habits have obviously become true addictions — drug addicts and alcoholics are the most obvious examples. But most unhealthy habits *are* addictions in the sense that we are caught up in them, and they control us more than we do them. *This is why people continue bad habits despite knowledge of the harmful, often lethal consequences.* In this sense, these habits are malignant, like untreated cancer. And like untreated cancer we often deny their seriousness. When using lethal drugs, for example, people talk about getting high, not about endangering their lives. To me, it is clear that whatever unhealthy habit we indulge in, we are, in some way, slowly or rapidly destroying ourselves — if not physically, then emotionally and spiritually. If it is not doing direct harm to our body, it is limiting our interactions with people and the rest of the world. Most important, practically everyone who has won out over an unhealthy habit or addiction feels better — life is richer, and they are more involved.

To illustrate the power of personal behavior, Table 10-1 lists six common health problems along with behaviors that will increase your chances of avoiding that problem. For example, regular seat belt use is a healthy habit that increases chances of avoiding injury in an auto accident. *What you do and don't choose to do now can make a big difference in your future health.* It is important to understand when you have a choice and what the consequences are.

TABLE 10–1.

Problems or Conditions	Healthy Habits
Injury or death from auto accident	Observing speed limits Wearing seat belts Not drinking alcohol or using drugs before or while driving
Infection and irritation of the throat and air passages	Not smoking Avoiding polluted areas
Liver problems	Not drinking alcohol to excess Not mainlining drugs Eating a balanced diet
Heart attack	Not smoking Checking blood pressure yearly Treating high blood pressure if present Eating carefully so as not to be overweight
Anxiety	Recognizing and expressing feelings Exercising regularly Regular spiritual activity
Unwillingness to change	Regular spiritual activity Reading Being open to criticism Regularly processing behavior with a friend or colleague Self-acceptance

WHAT ARE THE UNHEALTHY HABITS?

What are the unhealthy habits? You can probably name most of them as well as I can. Think about it a moment and write in your notebook what you think they are.

I define unhealthy habits as habitual behaviors that are self-destructive or limit growth in some significant physical or emotional-spiritual way. They may have immediate detrimental effects or more subtly appearing late aftereffects.

Here is a list of significantly unhealthy personal behaviors:

- lack of regular exercise
- overeating
- eating nutritionally poor or dangerous foods
- not wearing seat belts
- not brushing and flossing your teeth on a daily basis
- not having a yearly visit to the dentist for removal of tartar
- excessive use of caffeine
- smoking
- having more than two alcoholic drinks per day — some say five a week (a "drink" is one beer, one four-ounce glass of wine, or 1.5 ounces of hard liquor)
- too much sun exposure on bare skin
- habitual or compulsive use of "recreational drugs" or mood-altering substances
- unwillingness to consider change
- habitually acting or reacting out of fear

The first three habits in my list, lack of exercise, overeating, and eating nutritionally poor and dangerous foods, are all unhealthy habits of major significance. The next four chapters are devoted to them. Smoking, the abuse of alcohol and drugs, and failure to use seat belts are equally dramatic causes of death and disability. And smoking and substance abuse are not just problems for men. Due to increased smoking in recent decades, lung cancer now rates with breast cancer as the leading cause of death due to malignancy in women. Physicians are more likely to prescribe tranquilizers and other mood-altering chemicals to women than they are to men. With the cooperation of their physicians, many women become "pill junkies" to alleviate boredom, anxiety, depression, and low self-esteem. This is one of our most prominent public health problems.

In addition to the last three problems listed above, there are other destructive emotional habits. Automatic defensiveness is one. Isolation and withdrawal as a frequent behavior is also unhealthy. Talking incessantly and the inability to listen to others are other examples. The habit of being a victim (the victim mentality), or always blaming someone or something else thwarts growth for enormous numbers of people. Certain reactions to stress can be unhelpful. While more specific reference to these has already been made in the emotional-spiritual health chapters where they are discussed in more detail, the general principles that follow apply to emotional problems too.

Even if you are a long-time smoker, drink excessively, don't use seat belts, or never brush your teeth, there is hope that you can change. Many, many "hopeless" alcoholics have recovered with the help of Alcoholics Anonymous and other programs. Since the Surgeon General's report in 1964, 32,000,000 former smokers have stopped on their own. Drug addicts have beaten their habits through AA, other "twelve-step" programs like Narcotics Anonymous, and other drug treatment programs. Except in the case of people whose fundamental mental illness is so deep and pervasive that they are significantly out of touch with reality, there are few personal habits that are not potentially controllable.

Often, older people are characterized as "too old to change" or "set in their ways." Worse, part of our cultural folklore is that the proper activity of older folk is to sit around ruminating about the past and being content to continue behaving as they always have. If and when you get like this, is it because you choose to do so or because you feel that is what's ex-

pected? Remember, you may be excluding some exciting new adventures for yourself. You may be failing to refuel a still capable engine.

FOUR IMPORTANT CONSIDERATIONS

People wishing to change must heed the following considerations. They are more frequently neglected than not, and, as a result, attempts to change are often unsuccessful.

1. To be habitual is to forget there is a choice.
2. The personal benefits and meaning of the habit are critical to appreciate.
3. Change needs to be grieved.
4. A good support system is vital.

To Be Habitual is to Forget There is a Choice

To be habitual can be both good for you and bad for you. Choice is involved in both unhealthy and healthy habits. In unhealthy habits the choice often becomes unconscious. An addicted person behaves as if he or she has no choice. To change unhelpful habits requires a return to conscious choice. A helpful strategy for doing this is to think about your habit and write down all of the related choices you make every time you choose to indulge your habit.

Here is an example for smoking (though your choices might be a little different). When you choose smoking, you choose to do the one thing *known*, more than any other one thing, to increase risk for heart attack, *known* to be the causative agent in 90% of lung cancer (the most common U.S. cancer), *known* to be the causative agent in emphysema and chronic bronchitis, *known* to discolor teeth, make clothing smell and give breath that is unpleasant to all non-smokers (even former ones), *known* to decrease vitality and energy for living, *known* to decrease taste sensitivity, *known* to increase doctor's bills. That's what you choose.

The Personal Benefits and Meaning of the Habit are Critical to Appreciate

There is no habit, however harmful, that does not have important meaning or benefits to its owner. Every habit brings some benefit or has some important symbolic meaning to the inhabited person.

Look at some examples. The heroin user who is constantly lethargic and without feelings benefits from this kind of withdrawal. For whatever reason he or she benefits. The world may seem hostile, work too hard, or the boss too obnoxious. Many alcoholics enjoy (at least for a while) the release of inhibitions. They feel less shy and find it easier to talk to people, be assertive, or express that anger that's been smoldering. Alcohol can also provide a means of withdrawal, and some people use it (consciously and unconsciously) to help them sleep. Stimulation is another common benefit. A lot of people feel they are more creative when they drink alcohol or coffee, use drugs, or smoke. They believe their alertness and mental capability are increased. Large numbers of people use drugs, smoke, and drink to relax.

Thus, regardless of whether a habit is healthy or not, it provides benefits to the indulging person. It is vital to acknowledge this point, because too often people try to change habits without recognizing that they must get the same benefits in another way, or clearly and explicitly say goodbye to those benefits. If, for example, Chris benefits from alcohol by feeling more relaxed with his family, this is important and useful. But if his use of alcohol also results in belligerent behavior, he will need to find another way of relaxing with his family if and when he decides to stop drinking. If he doesn't, another source of stress is created.

All of the benefits that have been mentioned are ways of coping. However, they invariably have the effect of letting the person "out of life" instead of keeping them in. In even plainer language, they permit the user to withdraw or hide. They are a way of resisting change and remaining stuck. They require time and attention. They become parts of larger patterns that allow less and less time for other things. Wellness is a willingness to evolve and change, to forego one way of doing things in order to make way for something else — something that feels better day by day and brings real joy into life.

Take smoking again. It inhibits change by serving as an emotional shield. People holding cigarettes or pipes in their mouths with their hands are shielding themselves. The shielding prevents the expression of emotions in a normal or helpful way. It does this by distorting or hiding facial expressions. The cigarette, cigar, or pipe also becomes the center of attention so nuances of sensitivity in the cheeks and eyes, as well as the mouth are often missed entirely because of the observer's attention (or inattention) to the smoking object. One friend told me that the hardest thing for her about stopping smoking was that she felt so exposed. She couldn't hide behind her hand! Smoking also interferes with the reception of emotions. The smoker takes in smoke, he is preoccupied with keeping his smoke object lit, or in getting the next one. To whatever extent these things are happening, the smoker's intake channels are clogged. He cannot receive the messages.

Change Needs to be Grieved

A common mistake in controlling habits is failing to acknowledge that these habits must be grieved. Giving up cigarettes, alcohol, or drugs is a *major change*. An important aspect of the user's life is being abandoned. This involves very significant emotional adjustments.

The process of grieving is a health-giving process. When it is neglected, the consequences can be major and long lasting. As a young man and adolescent, my friend Bob had a close relationship with his dad. He followed him into the ministry but, over the course of several years, discovered that his own ideology and interests were not fulfilled by that vocation. He left the church and as a result became estranged with his father. There was appreciable anger and resentment on both sides. The loving and caring aspects of their relationship were gone. Bob was chronically depressed for several years. One day we were talking about his family (which at that time I knew little about) and this story came out. Inexplicably, as he talked, Bob became extremely flat and eventually began to sob. When this subsided he was in touch with a deep sadness and sense of loss about the positive aspects of his former relationship with his father. In all those years he had not effectively grieved the old loving relationship. After further exploration in a few sessions of therapy, his depression lifted entirely and has not returned.

Many people become depressed after giving up smoking, coffee, or alcohol. Sometimes it is true physical withdrawal, but it is often because the loss of the substance and its benefits are not grieved — there is no letting go. It is helpful to plan on grieving and to even schedule an event (a party or present to yourself) to acknowledge "officially" letting go.

A Good Support System is Vital

Numbers of people correct unhealthy habits without professional help. A recent article in *Psychology Today*[1] suggested that perhaps the majority of people who give up smoking or lose weight do so on their own or at least without a formal program or support group. However, there are still a lot of people around who want to change certain habits and seem

1. S. Schacter, "Don't Sell Habit-Breakers Short," *Psychology Today*, August 1982, p.27.

unable to do so at least on any permanent basis. My own bias is that more people would be successful if they did not try to do it on their own. (See Chapter 9 about support systems.) In no aspect of health is support more important than in trying to change habits. Unfortunately, it is an area where the "do it alone" behavioral pattern is very likely to take hold. We seldom get addicted alone—why believe we can get sober alone?

An additional dilemma is that people do not even think about the question of support until they are ready to change. Support systems can often be helpful in increasing someone's readiness to change. More of them can be used in that way. (See "On Doing it Alone," p. 95, in Chapter 9.)

AN APPROACH TO CHANGING A HABIT

The approach to changing habits involves four major steps. One, analyze the meaning and benefits of the habit in your life at the present time. Two, look at your life in terms of whether this is a good time to make a change. Three, decide to go ahead with the change (presuming the second step provides an affirmative answer). Four, mobilize and utilize the appropriate strategies and resources to make the change.

Analyzing Benefits and Meaning of Your Habit

If you have a habit that you'd like to give up or change significantly, try beginning with the following exercise. It is designed to help you perceive the benefits of your habit and to better understand how it functions as part of your whole being. Answer the following questions honestly and completely. Spend 15–20 minutes with them on one day and then an equal time the following day. It usually takes some incubation time to illuminate the important benefits and meanings.

1. What were the circumstances under which this habit got started? That is, during the period that it became fairly habitual, what factors and circumstances were present?
2. How will continuation or discontinuation of this habit relate to your health goals as stated in Chapter 2?
3. What are the benefits of this habit for you at the present time? Is it of value to you? What is that value? What is it doing for you? Does it help you hide and withdraw? Is it a stimulant and loosener for you? Does it do both kinds of things at different times or the same time?
4. What sort of problems is it creating for you (social, physical, emotional, on the job)?
5. Do you think it's part of a script, i.e., part of the reason you maintain this habit because your inner censors and controllers say that it is an important part of your image in the eyes of other people? What do you think would happen if your image changed in this particular way?
6. Considering all of the above, are there other ways in which you might derive the same benefits?
7. In what ways might you effectively grieve the loss of this habit?

There is nothing tricky or magic about this analysis. However, the more thought *and honesty* you can apply to these questions, the more helpful they will be. The answers to them will give you a much clearer view of how this habit functions for you, why it is important, and how much of that importance you can do without.

Fred, a chronically overweight and overeating 28-year-old person, answered these questions as follows:

1. As a child, my good behavior was rewarded with food. I received further praise for eating everything. Since my parents showed little love in other ways, I got to be a "good" and fairly constant eater. (My parents were both overweight too!)
2. One of my goals is to learn to eat normally and attain normal weight.
3. Now I think I still get a lot of attention by eating—I am "the garbage pail." I'm also praised for the treats I prepare and take to the office. I reward myself for other abstinence or "good behavior" with food.
4. No dates in two years. I hate myself and my looks. Just feel "fat" all the time.
5. Well, I think so. Yes, I certainly enjoy my reputation and the praise I get for the treats I take to the office. It's practically the only way I get praise.
6. I could continue to prepare treats — they don't have to be full of sugar and calories. With a little more practice, my work could improve to where I think it would make me proud — and praised. I might join a singing group. I've always had a good voice.
7. I could get my best friends together and say "goodbye" to Fred, the big eater, and all that goes with that. Talk about the benefits and really acknowledge them, but say goodbye.

Timing Your Change

The principal consideration here is how much is going on in your life. If you are under great pressure and stress and are undertaking other big changes, it may be better to wait. If you are involved in a divorce and your boss is new, that's probably enough change for the present. Wait a few months before giving up cigarettes.

Be careful, however, that you don't get in a rut where *now* is *never* the right time!

The Decision To Change

While a decision to change can obviously be made at any time, it will be more likely to succeed if you have done the analysis of benefit and meaning and decided that now is a good time. The decision should not be made lightly even if your habit has already been harmful to you. Nor should it be delayed for spurious reasons. Making the decision requires profound honesty. Don't deny! You are the only person qualified to make this decision. You can know yourself better than anyone else. The facts as you know them, your feelings about the habit and the situation, and your faith and spirituality must all come into play. If the change involves giving up a harmful activity, as contrasted with only starting a good habit, like flossing, which you don't do now, review your facts, feelings, and faith and then *give it some time.* The best course for you to take will soon become obvious.

Mobilizing Strategies and Resources

Find different ways of getting your benefits or acceptable alternative benefits. This is usually not hard to do but it is very important. Sometimes this is the substitution of a "positive addiction" (like exercise) for the unhealthy one you are trying to leave behind. Many have stopped smoking by becoming more and more addicted to exercise. Eventually they found their exercise was inhibited by their smoking, so they gave up the latter.

Plan a formal goodbye ceremony with friends, allies, fellow habiters, and those who have given up the habit. The ceremony can be humorous and sad. One simple but effective plan is to have each person reminisce about their association with you and the habit, how they liked you with the habit, and how they didn't. Then after some general discussion, do another round in which they speculate on how its going to be in the future, knowing you without your habit.

In the identification and mobilization of support, look around for allies, friends, family members, and groups who can support you wholeheartedly in this change. It is particularly important to ask (some people do this in writing) the support of those people who might (knowingly or unknowingly) subvert your effort to change. For example, one strategy used successfully in weight loss programs is to have each person in the group send out letters to the people they eat with on some regular basis. The letters explain what they are setting out to do, what their goals are, and ask for cooperation. More specifically, they ask that people not tease them about their effort and not try to persuade them to have "a little more of this or that because it's so good." Wherever possible, people are asked to eat the weight loser's food, rather than the weight loser having to prepare a special meal. If smoking is the habit in question, friends and associates are asked not to offer cigarettes, and, when possible, forego smoking in the person's presence. Look for groups in your neighborhood that are supporting the specific change you wish to make, e.g., Alcoholics Anonymous, Narcotics Anonymous, or stop-smoking groups. Every community will have some kind of group support. Some will be good, some bad, some free, some expensive. If there is not one for you, think about starting your own. (See Resources, Self-Help Group Consortium.)

In mobilizing support, do not forget whatever power you acknowledge as greater than yourself. If you believe in God or a Higher Power of any kind, ask for his/her/its support. Do it regularly and often. For a lot of people, this is the most helpful step of all.

Perhaps the single most important tool for many people is not to think back or ahead about your habit. Change for today and today only. "One day at a time" is all you need worry about. The psychological difference between moderating your eating, not smoking, or exercising *today,* and for the rest of your life is enormous. One day is manageable—a lifetime is not. Even a week or a month is usually not manageable. So do whatever it is you're going to do for today. Tomorrow will take care of itself.

Changing habits, particularly long-term ingrained ones, can be very difficult. It requires personal understanding, patience, commitment, faith, and a willingness to change. The benefits of the habit must be acknowledged, the change properly grieved, and a support system developed. Too many people try to change without clarity of choice and consequences. The important considerations of change and an approach to change have been outlined. These general principles apply to the change of almost any habit. Certainly they apply to the habits related to eating, body structure, and exercise, which are discussed in the next four chapters.

RESOURCES CHAPTER 10

Alcoholics Anonymous. The program which has helped countless alcoholics achieve sobriety. Few have recovered without AA. It is a spiritually inspired program of education in how to live so that alcohol is unnecessary. There are no rules, only guidelines. Everyone individualizes their program and proceeds at their own pace. Most communities have an AA listing in the phone book. Or call or write P.O. Box 459, Grand Central Station, New York, NY, 19917 (212) 686-1100.

Farquhar, J. *The American Way of Life Need Not be Hazardous to Your Health* (See General Resources). An invaluable aid to habit change. Gives specific and detailed strategies for exercise, stress management, weight management, and qualitative dietary change.

Heart Association. Local, State, and National Organizations. Have helpful information and programs regarding smoking, diets, exercise. Can sometimes provide speakers, always written materials.

Lung Associations—same as for Heart Associations.

Narcotics Anonymous, Overeaters Anonymous, and other so called "12-step programs" utilize the principles of AA. They also have local listings. National offices.

Ryan and Travis. *The Wellness Workbook* (General Resources). While the purpose of the workbook isn't specifically habit change, many of the exercises and strategies for wellness are useful for people trying to change their habits.

Seventh Day Adventists—in many states, the Seventh Day Adventists run stop-smoking programs that are short and significantly successful.

See also Resources for Chapter 9.

11

Healthy Body Structure Through Alignment, Flexibility and Muscle Balance

WHY a chapter on alignment, or — as it might also be called — posture? That's passé isn't it? And "flexibility"? How, you ask, do these relate to health? When I was young, I heard a lot about posture. "Sit up straight, Peter." "Don't slouch." As kids we were always comparing our muscles — showing how strong they were, but never how supple. I don't hear much about posture now but good alignment, flexibility, and balance are the first line of prevention against myriad pains, strains, backaches, and stiff necks. Alignment, flexibility, and balance are an important part of personal health competence. They can keep your muscles, joints, and spine free of pain and functioning well. When your body is aligned and flexible, you will feel at home in your body, using it gently and with respect.

When it comes to muscles and bones, medical doctors work on curing problems not on preventing them. "Minor" discomforts are treated with pills, heat, or both. The abnormalities of alignment and posture that can arise from them or be causing them are of no interest. Health maintenance with respect to structural problems is possible through attention to alignment and the proper use of your body as a biomechanical structure. Certain health practices prevent or minimize the possibility that you will get heart disease. In an analogous way, it is possible to minimize or prevent low back pain, shoulder pain, and other chronic muscle and joint problems by not misusing the body in your posture and tasks.

113

THE PLEASURE AND PAINS OF POSTURE

Assessing Your Alignment

To assess your alignment well, a full-length mirror is essential, and an interested friend can help you. Look at yourself in the morror while standing and sitting, from both the front and the side. Also, watch yourself in the mirror while you are walking, or look for your reflection in shop windows. As you make these assessments, honor your frame. Remember how well it *has* supported you over the years. Also, ask what you can do to help support yourself in a more relaxed, flowing, and functional way.

Facing the mirror directly, position your head as if you were looking at the horizon. Level your shoulders with one another and let them suspend from, rather than hold up, the neck. Is your pelvis level? Notice if you slump or become asymmetrical in some other way when you stand.

Now look at yourself from the side. The drawing in Figure 11-1 shows the normal curves of the spine and their relationships to one another. In some people the lower curve is exaggerated forward, and many have a more prominent backward curve in the thoracic part of the spine. Are your shoulders too far forward or back? Is the buttock tucked in? How is your abdomen? Does it stick out? If so, does that appear to be fatness or slackness of posture?

Pay attention to how fluid or tight you are in the ways you walk, run, make love. Look at your handedness: how fixed is it? Do you use either hand for simple tasks? Are your movement patterns fixed or variable? Do they tend to be always the same or are you creative?

Do this assessment over several weeks. Your sensitivity to your body will increase if you stay emotionally and spiritually connected. If you have pain or discomfort, spend time concentrating on it — don't "disconnect." Ask yourself what

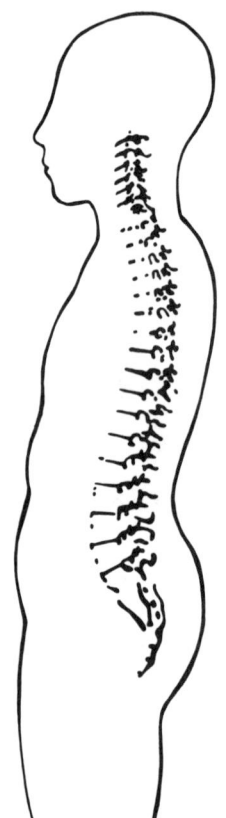

FIGURE 11–1   Normal Spine Curvature.

it means, why it has come now. Using pills for relief too soon or too regularly can result in disconnecting, whereas relief obtained from massage, heat, or pressure therapy will enhance your awareness.

Assuming and Maintaining Healthy Alignment

When assuming, improving, and/or maintaining healthy posture, two things are helpful. One is to picture your spine as a tent pole. The rest of the body flows down from it like a tent. This picture will help you let go of "holding the body up." The head is supported by the spine. The head and neck with attached muscles and connective tissue suspend the shoulders, trunk, and upper chest. The rest of the body is supported by the lower parts of the tent pole. Think of your body as being guided and supported from above.

Draw a picture of this and look at it every day. This is the "suspension mechanics" concept of body structure as contrasted with the "compression mechanics" concept that most of us have.

A second helpful idea for healthy alignment is a fantasy to help you guide and support your body from above. Find the point in the top of your head halfway between your ears. Pretend to screw a strong and painless hook into it. When working on your posture, imagine there is a strong rope attached to the hook which runs to a hot air balloon directly above (when standing) or slightly forward (when walking or running) of you. Feel it pulling gently upward on your head, then focus on your breath, and with each exhalation allow the release of tension. Try it, it works![1]

The next few paragraphs will describe healthy alignment for standing, sitting, and walking or running. They may feel awkward at first or may rarely cause discomfort in the lower back. If the suggested adjustments do not help, try consulting with someone knowledgeable in therapeutic yoga, or one of the bodywork specialists mentioned later in the chapter.

The concept of your body being guided and supported from above is central to good alignment whether you are sitting, standing, walking, or running. When standing, keep both feet firmly on the ground, toes slightly closer together than heels (awkward at first), with the weight transmitted through the inner (mostly) and outer (definitely) balls of your feet as well as through the heels. The feet can be together or apart, but distribute weight equally upon them. The knees should be straight but not locked. Tuck the buttocks in (forward), bring slight tension to the lower abdominal wall, level your shoulders and place them halfway between their most for-

ward and the most backward position into which they can be moved (the neutral position). Keep the head level so your eyes gaze directly forward at the horizon. As you become accustomed to these adjustments, your body will feel comfortable and you will feel strange when not in this position. If this posture causes discomfort in the lower back, try putting one foot in front of the other or one foot on a chair or step. If you do this, remember to change feet every five minutes or so.

When sitting, hold the body essentially the same as when standing from the pelvis on up. The buttocks and back of the thighs are planted equally on the sitting surface. The weight is on your buttock bones not your tailbone. Allow the hollow in the lower back to comfortably flatten. This can often be achieved by sitting with knees higher than hips. If back support is used evenly, distribute it throughout the lower half or mainly where the lowest ribs attach in the back. Again, level your shoulders, put them in the neutral position, and keep the head level. Don't cross your legs for long. If this is a compelling need due to inner tensions, try changing from side to side every five minutes or so. Postural asymmetries can develop from months and years of crossing legs more one way than the other.

Walk and run with the body inclined slightly forward from the ankles, not the waist. Think of your ankles as your earth hinge. The hook/rope/hot air balloon fantasy is also very helpful when walking or running. The balloon stays slightly in front of you to help you lean. The lean increases the faster you go. The effect is one of constantly falling forward, thus using gravity to help move ahead. Lots of people walk and run with their weight thrown backward. This requires more effort, puts undue strain on the lower back, and gives more jarring and concussion to the spine. With proper walking, other

1. I first heard this idea from Austin (Ozzie) Gontang of San Diego, CA.

body parts have the same relative positions as when standing. Keep your head level. Look down with your eyes only. Hold the arms fairly close to your sides. Let them swing naturally and relaxed. As your right leg goes forward your left arm goes forward, and vice versa. When running, flex your elbows comfortably, and as you stride, let your hands rotate in a vertical plane (like the pistons of a locomotive) parallel to the sides of your body. Keep the hands low.

The Posture of Lifting and Other Effort

Great damage can be done to the lower back and other parts of the spine by improper lifting. An inflexible frame can accelerate and accentuate this. The cardinal rule when lifting is to keep the lower spine as straight as possible. Even when you bend your knees correctly, you will sometimes need to bend forward from the line of the pelvis and hips. This is okay and is different from bending the lower spine either backward (thereby exaggerating the hollow) or forward, creating a curve which is opposite to the usual curve. So, keep the lower (lumbar and sacral) spine as nearly straight as possible when lifting *anything*; a lot of backs "go out" when lifting an insignificant weight. *Do not bend your lower spine forward or backward while lifting.* Bend your knees and lift by straightening your legs again. It may look strange but it is a lot healthier.

A dangerous activity for the back is shoveling, particularly snow. Wet snow is heavy, and the lever arm of the shovel puts much greater strain on the spine than if you lifted the same snow from a place beneath your feet. It is not easy to follow the straight spine rule while shoveling but it really pays to find ways of doing it. Always keep one foot in front of the other. Do not reach forward. Focus on bending your knees and ankles. A short (15–18 inch) piece of rope attached to the neck of the shovel with a loop for your hand helps immensely. If available, a snowblower is better.

Various sports are asymmetrical because they put unequal stress on the two sides of the body. Tennis, golf, bowling, and racquetball are examples. Over the years, they can cause problems in the neck, back, shoulders, and arms. If you play these games frequently, it is important to warm up and cool down using a symmetrical routine (see Appendix C). It is also good for unilateral exercisers to take up a second exercise which is bilateral, such as running, walking, swimming, or cycling.

FLEXIBILITY AND MUSCLE BALANCE

What is meant by flexibility and muscle balance? Why work for it? A body (no matter how large or small, long or short, fat or thin) that is flexible and balanced is a healthy, competent body. By flexible, I mean tuned but supple, lithe and longer, not tight and hard. Muscle balance is the appropriate difference, or non-difference, between the tone and strength of opposing muscle groups, like those in front of the thigh versus those behind the thigh and those above the knee versus those below the knee.

If you are a muscular person, it is even more desirable to maintain flexibility. Whatever you wish to do, you will do it better. If you are a runner, cycler, swimmer, skier, or rope skipper, flexibility and muscle balance is essential to avoid or minimize injury. This is also true of activities involving sudden movements and bursts of speed like basketball, tennis, racquetball, football, heavy labor, and sexual activity. Many injuries in either conditioning or fast action sports begin with muscle spasm or cramping, or involve sudden or repeated strain on a joint. Many stress ("overuse") injuries in runners (tendonitis, plantar fascitis, shin splints) are caused or increased by imbalances between the front and back muscles in the legs. Many joint problems are not from trauma to the joints themselves but from improper flexibility and muscle balance above and below the problem spot. Maintaining flexibility will minimize muscle spasm, and maintaining the right balance of muscular tone and strength around a joint will allow it to function properly and lessen its potential for injury.

With good flexibility and muscle balance, your body will also feel better. It will be looser and more open, and you will be correspondingly more open as a person.

Flexibility is attained by stretching. An effective, safe stretch elongates the fleshy parts of the muscles. Most good stretches need to last 30–60 seconds — this I'll call a "major stretch." Ease into the stretch while breathing smoothly, but don't overbreathe. After 15–20 seconds go as fully into the stretch as possible. You may feel mild burning pain or soreness but should not feel tearing or sharp pain. Continue to breathe regularly, even when doing abdominal and back stretches. After a total of 30–60 seconds ease out of the stretch. Don't stop suddenly. Relax completely before beginning the next stretch. DO NOT BOUNCE IN ANY STRETCH, as it can be harmful.

Stretching exercises are most effective when you exhale *through* the structures being stretched. For example, if stretching your calf, concentrate on "breathing out" through the calf. This is a basic part of yoga technique, and it is not difficult to learn, although it may sound crazy. As you end each stretch, relax for 10–20 seconds, *particularly* the stretched part. Continue to concentrate on your breathing, but now focus on your chest or on the movement of air through your nostrils.

Balance between opposing muscle groups is achieved by flexibility with strengthening certain muscles. Running shows why muscle balance is important. The power in running comes primarily from the back muscles of the upper and lower leg, the buttocks, and low back — the "posterior" muscles. This is particularly true of level running; hills strengthen the anterior leg muscles also. If measures are not taken to stretch these power muscles well and to strengthen and tone the muscles in front of the leg, muscle imbalance occurs and injuries result.

A Routine for Maintaining Flexibility/Muscle Balance

The routine described in Appendix C is one way of attaining and maintaining good flexibility and appropriate balance between opposing muscle groups. It is a combination of major stretches, some maintained longer than others, and repetitive movements. The latter provide strength to certain muscle groups or increase mobility of certain joints, or both. There are many other routines for attaining the same or greater flexibility. One of them is to become a disciplined practitioner of hatha yoga, which is discussed in Chapter 20. If you are already practicing yoga regularly you probably don't need to do anything else for flexibility and muscle balance.

The program described in the appendix will assure flexibility and muscle balance for running, swimming, bicycling, or almost any sustained and vigorous aerobic program. To the extent of present knowledge, it is safe, particularly for the back. It involves attending explicitly to each of the following groups of muscles and the related joints: neck, shoulders and arms, low back and buttocks, abdomen, front of the legs, and the back of the legs. Everyone may want to emphasize some areas of the body more than others and will probably want to add modifications or stretches of their own.

STRUCTURAL PROBLEMS AND INJURIES

"Bad" backs, painful necks, and other muscular aches and pains are common. They vary from mild but nagging discomforts to dramatic disabling events. Physicians take care of these problems but most are not very good at it. We do reasonably well with an acute joint injury or a fracture, but when it comes to back and neck problems and other assorted muscular ailments, we usually prescribe heat and aspirin or a tranquilizer, say we don't know why it's happened, and hope it will go away. Most doctors consider these problems uninteresting.

Like other discomforts, pain arising from the musculoskeletal structures is trying to tell us something. It may be a matter of life-style, tension at work or home, doing too much, or even being bored. It may also mean that the person is structurally injured. When a football player pulls a hamstring during a sudden cut or acceleration, no one questions that there is an injury. Less well accepted by doctors and lay people alike is that many injuries are generated over months or years by poor posture, lack of flexibility, or misuse of the body in some repetitive way.

The basic trauma in such instances can be a frequently used abnormal posture (like sitting, standing, walking) or one that is used infrequently but generates greater forces (lifting, shoveling, running). Such injuries and their chronic compensatory change can alter alignment and supporting structures, impinge on nerves, and affect body image.

JOE'S STORY

When I first met Joe he had been working for some time as a paramedic and fireman.

He was 35 and for years had experienced recurrent low back pain which was sometimes severe enough to make work difficult and inhibit his sailing, a favorite pastime. I showed him some low back strengthening and stretching exercises, which helped significantly. He then had long periods relatively free of pain, despite lifting, sailing, sex, and his work. About two years ago, Joe became quite serious about running. As his commitment increased, his enjoyment and mileage grew, but he was limited by increasingly severe and tenacious back pain. When he ran more than 15 miles a week, the pain returned and the exercises did less good. After massage and additional exercise failed to change anything, he went to an osteopath. The evaluation showed that Joe's right leg was a quarter of an inch shorter than the left. A week after inserting a lift in his right running shoe, Joe had no further discomfort while running, and it has not returned. His back is essentially pain free the rest of the time as well.

A difference in leg length of one-quarter inch is not always enough to produce symptoms in someone with normal activity. But a running program (or another strenuous and repetitive activity) can create enough additional trauma to cause or increase symptoms. Joe's lift restored the symmetry needed to provide relief.

As with other injuries, the body tries to heal those of alignment and posture. But since the basic cause is chronic and repetitive (i.e., the poor alignment), the injury continues or is aggravated. Compensation becomes a major part of the healing process; for example, the spine may curve another way or additional connective tissue may be laid down to guard an area that is painful with movement. This extra tissue or new curvature allows more function at first, but paradoxically causes further postural abnormality, local irritation, or sets up a weakness, any of which may behave later as a more serious injury.

The Lower Back

The frequency of low back pain suggests that perhaps homo sapiens has not yet found the best posture for our frame!

Avoidance of back pain and successful treatment of it are matters of following the suggestions already made with respect to standing, sitting, walking, running, lifting, and shoveling. There are also healthy sleeping guidelines. A very firm mattress or a thin pad on a carpeted floor are the most comfortable sleeping surfaces. There are two healthy positions. The first is on the side with knees bent and drawn up slightly toward the head. The top knee can be drawn up farthest and supported by a pillow. The second is on the back with a pillow or small bolster under the knees. Sleeping on the stomach, or on the back without knees slightly elevated tends to exaggerate that lumbar hollow we talked about, putting unfavorable strain on the lower back, and the neck, too.

If you are already having back pain, the suggestions for good alignment should be followed. In addition, do the exercises designated for the low back in the flexibility and muscle balance routine (Appendix C). If you are diligent and still have no relief, get help from your physician, a person skilled in therapeutic yoga, or one of the body-work people mentioned later in this chapter.

If not from muscle spasm or an injured muscle or ligament, low back pain often comes from disease of the shock absorbing spinal disks between the round spinal bones (the vertebral bodies). In response to sudden or repeated trauma (including those of stressful postures), the fibrous bands that hold the cushioning material between the vertebral bodies can degenerate or weaken and eventually rupture. The semi-solid material leaks out and may put pressure on one or two spinal nerves on their way to the pelvis and legs. This can give pain or weakness in certain muscle groups in the adjacent back, the buttocks, or part of the leg.

A "disk problem" is serious and should be professionally evaluated, but it is not always obvious when low back pain is due to a disk and when it is not. Postures or movements which exaggerate the lumbar curve or result in its curving very far the other way (hyperflexion) — like touching the toes with the knees straight, and certain yoga postures (see Chapter 20) — are potentially damaging to the disk.

The Neck Shoulders, and Upper Back

Like the lower part of the spine, the upper one is also vulnerable to injury. Those body parts connected to the upper spine by bone, muscle, or nerve are prone to tension, pain, and discomfort. The trapezius muscle running from the top of the shoulder blade to the base of the neck on either side is especially susceptible. The trouble can range from a "frozen neck" with incredible pain on slight movement to mild muscle aching and stiffness. While sudden movements, strenuous work, and injuries can often be implicated as the cause, more often than not there is no clear-cut physical cause. Emotional factors play a major role.

I recently had an injury where physical trauma and emotional-spiritual factors were both important. Away from home on several days of business, I was, in addition, determined to settle an old racing score between myself and a good friend. We had enjoyed a friendly but serious running rivalry for several years. The last time we raced he had beaten me soundly. For two years prior to this trip I had not raced because I was trying to understand why it seemed so important to me to compete and be successful. I had made considerable progress. However, when this trip to the friend's hometown loomed on the horizon, my "work" of the prior two years moved into the background. I made plans to race without considering its implications in terms of what I had been trying to accomplish.

The day before we were to race, I was running in an unfamiliar place when my foot caught in a loop of unseen tree root. I flew into the air and landed with a crash, spread-eagled on my outstretched hands, feet, and knees. It shook me up considerably but after a brief rest I felt no ill effects and completed my run. The next morning while doing pushups I noticed pain in my left trapezius muscle. It felt like many minor spasms I have easily massaged out and stretched away. Not this time! Over a few hours this spasm progressed to involve the back and top of my shoulder girdle, the entire trapezius muscle, and the muscles along the left side of the neck. The pain was intense. I essentially could not move.

It took a couple of weeks and two 1½ hour visits to an osteopath before I was really comfortable again. It was several days before I could run. The race was not held. The osteopath and I think that the fall plus the inner tension between my ego wanting to race and my more integrated self wanting to continue the "work" of the previous few months combined to produce the freeze. "Coincidence" and my mind-body connections had combined to keep me noncompetitive at least a little longer.

Prevention of neck/shoulder/upper back difficulties depends on avoiding acute injury or chronic abuse, and in becoming aware of emotional reaction patterns that may trigger pain. Prevention also involves keeping the muscles and body structures aligned through good posture, toned and flexible through an exercise and muscle balance routine, and balanced through equal use of the two sides of the body.

In understanding the importance of the latter, watch people going about their daily tasks. Notice how asymmetrically many operate with respect to their upper body. The business man walking to work with the heavy briefcase (most people carry them more often with one hand than the other), the woman holding her baby, the teenager or college student going to class with a knapsack draped over one shoulder, the laborer shoveling all day from the same side of his body, the waiter or waitress repeatedly carrying the tray in the same hand. These are all asymmetrical postures. When repeated for months or years, they can alter alignment and balance significantly. Compensatory malalignments in adjacent structures occurs with subsequent spasm, pain, and chronic injury.

WHO CAN HELP WITH YOUR STRUCTURE

If you are having problems with your body or are interested in a program of structural body health, there are sources of expertise and support. Yoga must be classed among the best of these. With the right instructor (it is hard to learn good yoga using only a book), a person can correct poor alignment while simultaneously developing strength, flexibility, and balance. It is hard work, however, and may take a long time. Yoga is further discussed, including precautions, in Chapter 20 as an alternative therapy.

Also among the foremost options are various kinds of body-work; several are exellent for promoting structural integrity and preventing its decline. Rolfing (developed by Dr. Ida Rolf) and Soma Neuro-Muscular Integration (developed by Dr. Bill Williams and Dr. Ellen Gregory) are deep tissue therapies designed to create more complete structural integrity. Working with the connective tissues and muscles these approaches are capable of altering the structural compensation that occurs as a result of injury or emotional trauma. As an additional benefit they are able to increase biomechanical efficiency by balancing opposing muscle groups.

The Alexander technique is a gentle form of movement education focused primarily on the relationship of the head and neck and their influence on the rest of the body. It has helped many dancers and athletes learn to use their bodies in a more functional way. The Feldenkreis school teaches ways of heightening self-awareness through movement. The movements and subtle exercises actually create structural change.

Illana Rubenfeld has created the Rubenfeld Synergy method by blending the Alexander technique, the movement awareness exercises of Feldenkreis, and the gestalt techniques of Fritz Perls. Her therapeutic approach incorporates vivid imagery and light touch techniques as well as movement training.

Osteopathy and chiropractic are usually applied to obvious problems, although they have excellent health maintenance potential as well. By manipulating musculoskeletal structures, they re-establish the integrity and alignment of acutely or chronically injured tissues. Osteopaths have the training and perspectives of MDs in addition to their knowledge and skill in manipulation. They believe that subtle (as well as major) structural abnormalities can be a significant cause of pain and dysfunction. Osteopaths trained in the last 20 years tend to use manipulation less and less. This is unfortunate since lots of physicians treat with medicines and surgery and few are skilled in manipulation.

Much to my relief, both chiropractors and osteopaths seem to be doing more "low force" manipulation and less "high velocity" stuff, like "cracking" necks. I am personally frightened by some high velocity work involving sudden forceful movements of body parts, particularly for neck problems. I would discourage it unless you have had it done before and feel that it is helpful.

Body alignment, flexibility, and muscle balance are the basic ingredients of structural health. When they are attained and maintained, a person's vulnerability to both serious musculoskeletal problems and the more common nagging muscular aches and pains (of Anacin fame) are greatly diminished. The techniques required to do this are not difficult and do not require fancy or expensive equipment, only a modicum of time and that warrior of all health activities — discipline.

The next chapter is on physical conditioning through exercise. Anyone doing regular and vigorous exercise is vulnerable to injury. The practices discussed in this chapter for maintaining alignment, flexibility, and muscle balance must be practiced to prevent eventual injury.

RESOURCES CHAPTER 11

Bodywork Organizations:
1. Soma Neuro-Muscular Integration: developed by Dr. Bill Williams and Dr. Ellen Gregory. Practitioners in your area may be located by writing Soma Practitioner's Association, 10798 SW 46th St., Miami, Florida, 33165, or by calling Dale Alexander (305) 449-5903.
2. Structural Integration (Rolfing): developed by Dr. Ida Rolf. Contact the Rolf Institute, 302 Perl, Boulder, Colorado, 80302 (303) 449-5903.
3. Information on Bonnie Pruden's methods of rehabilitation can be obtained by writing to 1 Elon Street, Stockbridge, MA 01262 (617) 298-3781. She has also written a book, *Pain Erasure: The Bonnie Pruden Way.* New York: Ballantine, 1982.
4. *Feldenkreis Guide*, P.O. Box 11145, Main Office, San Francisco, CA 94107.

Benjamin, B. *Sports Without Pain.* New York: Summit Books, 1979.

Bloom, M. "Meet the Manipulators," *American Health*, Vol. 2, #3, 1983 p. 68. Compares chiropractors, osteopaths, and orthopedic surgeons, particularly with respect to their management of back problems.

Franklin, N. "Bodywork: It Does a Body Good," *Medical Self-Care*, #34, Spring, 1984. Compares Movement Reeducation (Alexander and Feldenkreis) with Deep Tissue Manipulation (Rolfing) and Meridian based energy therapies (shiatsu, reflexology) and some combination styles.

Hitu, J. *Surviving Exercise*. New York: Houghton Mifflin, 1963.

12

Body Movement and Conditioning

"How much happiness is gained and how much misery escaped, by frequent and violent agitation of the body."

SAMUEL JOHNSON

WHY EXERCISE

Some kind of body movement and exercise is essential to higher levels of health competence. Not only is it valuable for its direct effects on body and mind, but it also enriches whatever else one does to be health competent. This chapter is aimed primarily at people contemplating a conditioning program or those who have started one and are still tentative and full of questions. It is for the person who is becoming health competent and chooses to make exercise a part of that process.

The benefits of exercise, and in recent years running in particular, have been greatly proclaimed and exalted. Here is a summary of the most important benefits. First, even without great change in physical prowess, a regular exercise program enhances body fitness and self-image. Moving the muscles, joints, and blood around is to the psyche like air is to a sagging tire. It provides energy, self-sufficiency, and often spiritual awareness. Realizing you have the competence to walk five or run two miles without undue strain provides a new sense of freedom.

Second, although there is a real decline of fitness potential with age, we are learning from older athletes that when fitness is maintained year by year, the decline in potential is much slower than we thought (and than our cultural norms teach us). So, as shown in Figure 12-1, people who exercise regularly over the years maintain abilities at or near their full potential, while those who do not exercise regularly are not only in poor condition but lose a lot of that potential.

Related to this is the fact that the older a person the more protection vigorous exercise provides from death due to coronary artery disease (the most common cause of heart attack). For people in their forties, heavy exercise decreases a person's risk for death from heart attack by 32 percent. For those in their seventies, heavy exercise decreases that risk by 66 percent.

Third, as people age, there is a cultural tendency to move the body less. *And as we move it less, we are able to use it less.* When joints and their surrounding muscles are not used, tone, strength, and flexibility are lost. These qualities maintain normal joint alignment and protect them from strain and injury. Without tone, strength, and flexibility, structures are not optimally maintained and injury occurs (see Chapter 11). Over time, the joint becomes damaged or inflexible, and the cycle is repeated. When arthritis (like rheumatoid arthritis or degenerative ar-

thritis) is present, this tendency is exaggerated. I believe that a significant part of the decline in joint usefulness in rheumatoid as well as other kinds of arthritis is caused by disuse, not by the severity of the disease itself.

Fourth, and perhaps most importantly, regular exercise is the best way to keep in touch with our body. To many, this may sound mystical and "far out." If so, that's primarily because for many, it is an unknown experience to be really in touch with their bodies. For most of us, our house or apartment is a place that we are "in touch with." We certainly are aware of fluctuations in temperature (sometimes of as little as one degree), of changes in air flow, lighting, the need for cleaning, painting, repairs, and replacements. However, people are not nearly as in touch with their bodies as with their houses — to say nothing of the differences in the resources that people spend on house maintenance as opposed to body maintenance.

Several other benefits of regular exercise include the following.

- Improved blood circulation throughout the body.

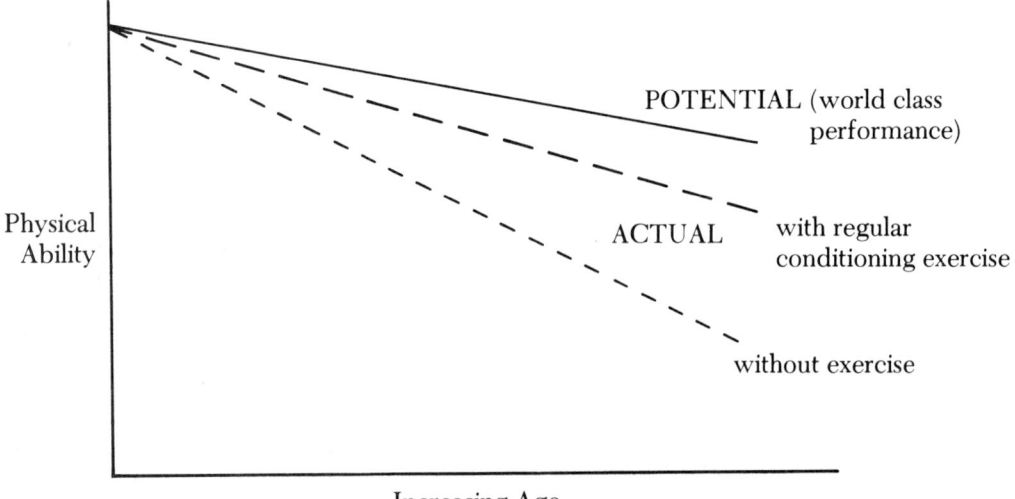

FIGURE 12-1   Exercise and Physical Ability.

- More efficient working together of lungs, heart, and muscles.
- Increased "good" (high-density) cholesterol in the blood, which counteracts the unhealthy effects of "bad" (low-density) circulating cholesterol.
- Helps an individual to handle stress, so he or she works more effectively.
- Improved psychological well-being, bolstering enthusiasm and optimism.
- Enhanced personal appearance. It releases tension and helps relaxation and sleep.
- Along with a balanced diet, it helps control weight.
- Conditioned people tire less easily.

THE DIFFERENT EFFECTS OF EXERCISE

Regular exercise can do three principal things for the body:

1. Increase flexibility, muscle balance, and relaxation of joints, tendons, and muscles.
2. Condition the heart, lungs, and skeletal muscles for stamina and endurance (fitness).
3. Increase strength, definition, and sometimes size of muscles and muscle groups.

An exercise program that is health competent will provide both flexibility and balance and aerobic fitness. Flexibility and muscle balance can only be achieved through a regular stretching routine. This is further discussed in the previous chapter and in Appendix C. There are many activities that provide aerobic conditioning. Practically all of them will also improve muscular strength and definition in the legs (walking, running, cycling, skating, jazzercise), and some will strengthen the upper body as well (swimming, ballet, gymnastics, rope jumping, cross-country skiing, some manual labor and heavy construction). Weight lifting, although excellent for muscle building, is seldom effective as an aerobic conditioner.

The rest of this chapter is devoted to conditioning for stamina and endurance, i.e., aerobic fitness. *Aerobic* is a term used by physiologists and biochemists meaning *with oxygen*. Aerobic exercise uses oxygen steadily for long periods. It provides healthful conditioning for the heart, lungs, and muscles and improves blood flow to those organs. A conditioned person can go for long periods at a steady pace (which is below his or her maximum pace for that exercise), while an unconditioned person of the same age, sex, and body build will tire very quickly at a much slower pace. There are also *anaerobic* sports which use little or no oxygen and can only be done for short periods. Fast sprints in track and swimming under water without scuba gear or snorkel are examples. Still other athletics, like basketball, racquetball, and tennis, are both anaerobic and aerobic.

LOOKING AT YOUR EXERCISE AND ACTIVITY PATTERNS

As a first step in assessing your own activity levels and patterns, complete the chart shown in Figure 12-2. This will also help: 1) make an estimate of caloric expenditure through exercise; 2) identify ways in which you can increase conditioning through everyday activities; 3) help identify barriers (psychological, financial, logistic) to making or increasing your commitment to exercise.

There can be considerable overlap between normal living activities, those considered recreational, and those that are part of a conditioning program. A laborer may be conditioned through his daily work. Certainly most bicyclers, runners, and swimmers (as well as others) consider their exercise both recreational and conditioning. In filling out the chart, put each activity in only one category.

FIGURE 12-2   Personal Exercise Profile.

Personal Exercise Profile

Circle any of the following activities which you do regularly	Estimate minutes spent at each circled activity each week	Write in any benefits you receive from the activity (Examples: stress reduction, fitness, creativity)	List any barriers that keep you from doing the conditioning, and flexibility and balance activities (this may not apply to you); Examples: time, not interested, no one to do it with
Routine Exercise			
Walk to work, store, etc.			
Walk upstairs			
Job requires exercise			
Lawn care/gardening			
Scrubbing/housework			
Others (Name)			
Recreational Exercise			
Team sports, such as basketball, volleyball, etc.			
Individual competitive sports, such as tennis, handball, etc.			

Non-competitive sports, such as hiking, skiing, biking, etc.

Dancing

Others (name) _____

Fitness program

Bicycling, swimming, cross-country skiing

Jogging, running, jumping rope, etc.

Calisthenics

Special Exercises

Aerobic dancing (jazzerobics, jazzercise)

Stretching

Yoga

Others (name) _____

Fill out the benefits column. Think about each activity in your list in terms of the potential benefits to you. Don't forget that benefits are not necessarily all physical! Finally, think of the barriers that prevent you from doing some regular recreational or conditioning exercise.

BARRIERS TO EXERCISE

People create reasons for not beginning or staying involved in exercise programs. It is important that people who are having trouble getting started or even those who are merely contemplating a program give consideration and discussion to these impediments. Some are more often excuses than valid reasons for not getting involved.

Time is given as the commonest barrier to exercise—"I don't have time." We ride in cars and elevators rather than walk to save time. We can't take time for morning exercises. We can't get away for a regular tennis game or a hike with the family. Actually time is probably more a symbol for inertia, a convenient excuse than an actual barrier. With the additional energy that comes as the result of regular exercise and with the time saved from sleep (most people need less if they exercise regularly), a program does not require extra time.

A second barrier to exercise is that we're "just too tired." At the end of a tense day, we want to plop down and relax, even though a swim or a game of ball would probably help relax us and restore our energy. Once you begin, this barrier will reverse; it will take care of itself.

Embarrassment is another difficult barrier for many people. Those in poor condition are often afraid that others will make fun of them. They're embarrassed at their appearance, their abilities, or both.

Another significant barrier is the lack of someone to exercise with. This is crit-

ical in competitive sports and is a real disadvantage in developing a regular exercise pattern around team activities.

Weather can also be a barrier, particularly for the person who is limited to a specific sport or outdoor activity. Regular skiing or ice skating in the winter must be combined with summer sports for a year-round program.

The fear of doing oneself harm is another barrier. People are afraid they may have heart attacks, break a hip, suffer a stroke. If you start with a realistic program (depending on your initial degree of fitness) and progress slowly, exercise will always be beneficial, even if you are chronically ill to begin with. A lot of this fear is engendered by physicians who fear malpractice if anyone has a problem.

In women, regular exercise can be associated with menstrual irregularities and infertility. Infrequent or absent bleeding, or greatly reduced flow in regularly spaced periods are the commonest examples of the former. The exact mechanisms are unknown but low body fat, alterations in endocrine function, and qualitatively poor nutrition are thought to be involved. Usually a decrease in the amount of exercise or an increase in weight, or both will result in a return to normal. It should not be assumed that all menstrual irregularity in exercising women is related to the exercise.

IMPROVING FITNESS THROUGH EVERYDAY ACTIVITIES

Despite the fitness boom, our society is still sedentary. We travel by car or public transport to work, to shop, and often to attend our recreation and exercise! Exercise for most of us is not integrated into the rest of our lives. Able people take the elevator up one or two floors. Others drive up and down in supermarket parking lots to get a few yards closer to the entrance or drive five or six blocks to get an ice cream cone. By itself, any one of these things won't keep you out of shape, but together they add up.

Routine daily activities can provide substantial conditioning effects. A person can stay in good condition by walking or bicycling instead of riding, climbing stairs instead of taking the elevator, using a hand-powered lawn mower and sawing firewood by hand. To illustrate the effectiveness of this, there are four small isolated population groups in the world whose people commonly live more than 100 years. Although the groups have many things in common one of the most singular is that they all get a lot of exercise which is integrated into their daily activities. They walk, run, do manual labor, and thereby exercise most of the day. While such a pattern is not feasible for many of us, it is possible to move significantly closer to it than the way we live now.

You can creatively increase your exercise during an average day in many ways. I have a friend who bicycles 12 miles round-trip to work two or three times a week, climbs the stairs to his ninth-floor office two to three times each day, and walks to the grocery store on a consistent basis. Here is a list of tricks you can use.

- Take stairs instead of elevator
- Walk between stores
- Walk to work
- Park at far end of the parking lot or several blocks from the office
- Get off the bus one or more stops too soon
- Do extra housework (mopping, vacuuming)
- Mow the lawn instead of hiring a teenager (and do it by hand)
- Garden (extra sweeping, hoeing, digging)
- Bicycle to stores or to work
- Walk down the hall to talk to colleagues instead of using the office phone
- Walk to eating place at lunch

It is possible to burn an additional 300–2000 calories a week by simple changes in everyday patterns. By walking upstairs to his office (9th floor, two or three times a day), my friend uses 400–600 calories a week. That's like running 250–300 miles a year!

EVERYBODY'S EXERCISE

As kids we all moved around on our feet a lot—walked, ran, shuffled. For many of us that stopped when we got our driver's license. But walking is now on the rise again. Thousands of people are enjoying the benefits of this practically non-traumatic exercise.

There is enough fitness-era experience with walking to suggest that people stick with it because it is relatively free of injury, and there is more time to enjoy the scenery and companions. It's certainly cheap. It can be aerobic if done briskly enough. Consistent walking workouts have favorable effects on the serum cholesterol fractions (may not lower your cholesterol but it will increase the high density to low density ratio) and decrease the propensity for clotting to occur in your blood vessels. Many think it improves their ability to remember things and think clearly. It definitely burns calories. An hour's brisk walk uses the same number of calories as a four-mile run.

Perhaps most important, it has good effects psychologically, helping to relieve anxiety, tension, and flat or mildly depressed moods. If you let it, it will also improve your sense of humor, even let you laugh at yourself once in a while. You know, feel like a kid again!

Getting Prepared for a Regular Fitness Program

Getting prepared requires three steps: 1) checking your health status; 2) learning to take your pulse; and 3) understanding target zones for heart rate.

The question that is asked most often, particularly by older people, is, "How do I know that it is okay for me to begin a fitness program?" The following questionnaire is one way to find out. If you answer "no" to every question and if your blood pressure is normal, experience has shown that no further screening is required for people up to 40 years of age. *This does not mean that you are immune to heart attack.* It does mean that you are probably as safe beginning a gradual exercise program, utilizing the steps outlined in the following pages, as you are conducting your usual daily activities. If your answer to one or more of the questions is "yes," consult your physician or an exercise specialist *before* beginning an exercise program or taking a fitness (stress) test.

Yes   *No*

_____ _____ 1. Has your doctor ever said you have heart trouble?

_____ _____ 2. Do you frequently have pains in your heart and chest?

_____ _____ 3. Do you often feel faint or have spells of severe dizziness?

_____ _____ 4. Has a doctor ever said your blood pressure was too high?

_____ _____ 5. Has your doctor ever told you that you have a bone or joint problem such as arthritis that has been aggravated by exercise or might be made worse with exercise?

_____ _____ 6. Is there a good physical reason not mentioned here why you should not follow an activity program even if you wanted to?

_____ _____ 7. Are you over age 65 and not accustomed to vigorous exercise?

_____ _____ 8. Did either of your parents have a heart attack before the age of 60?

_____ _____ 9. Are you taking any heart or blood pressure medications? If yes, what is its name?

Measuring Your Heart Rate

Since your heart is vitally involved in aerobic conditioning, you must learn to monitor the speed at which it beats by taking your pulse before, during, and after exercise. The method for taking your pulse is described in Chapter 5.

To obtain an exercise heart rate, count the pulse for ten seconds, then multiply the results by six to give the pulse in beats per minutes. When you count the pulse, keep your fingers on the artery and feel for regularity. Does the pulse speed up or slow down or skip beats? Record the rate and regularity.

Target Range for Your Pulse During Exercise

Now you need to understand the concept of the *target range* for pulse rate. By elevating your pulse into the target range, you can achieve effective conditioning with minimal risk. The longer you keep your heart rate in this range during a workout, the more effective the conditioning. Exercise that elevates your pulse into this range and enables you to keep it there for a period of 30 minutes or longer, three times a week or more, will after several weeks result in very effective conditioning. In order to avoid damage to feet, legs, and perhaps the heart as well, a beginner must work up to both the 30-minute period and the target heart zone gradually over five to eight weeks. Exercise that increases your pulse to levels under the target range is beneficial, but it will not condition you to the same degree. As you get older, attention to the target zone is more important for reasons of safety. Sustained exercise over the target limits may fatigue and even damage the heart. The older a person is, the more likely this is to happen.

TABLE 12–1 Exercise Target Zones.

Age	Maximum	Exercise Target Range
	Heart Rate	
10	210	147–179
15	205	144–174
20	200	140–170
25	195	137–166
30	190	133–162
35	185	130–158
40	180	126–153
45	175	123–149
50	170	119–145
55	165	116–140
60	160	112–136
65	155	109–132
70	150	105–128

Find the age closest to your own on the left. Your exercise target range for heart rate is then found on the right.

Table 12-1 gives the lower and upper limits of target zone according to age in years. The lower and upper limits of the zone are 70 and 85 percent, respectively, of the *calculated maximal rate* for a given individual. The calculated maximal rate is obtained by subtracting your age from 220. *Actual* maximal heart rates vary and can only be measured during a treadmill or bicycle stress test.

Choosing the Right Exercise

1. Pick an activity you consider *fun.*
2. Start with activities that do not in-

volve a lot of trouble and paraphernalia (logistically speaking).
3. Something you can do alone *or* with someone else is best.

Jogging or running, swimming, bicycling, skipping rope, and cross-country skiing are all good aerobic exercises. As previously stated, walking is wonderful, and it can be an effective aerobic conditioner if done briskly and for long enough. See Table 12-2.

TABLE 12–2 Approximate Calorie Consumption per Minute of Various Activities

Walking	(3 miles/hr)	4.0
Bicycling	(10 miles/hr)	6.0
Swimming	(1.5 miles/hr)	7.5
Running	(7.5 miles/hr)	12.5
Rope Jumping		6.0
Golf	(18 holes, no cart)	2.0

These values are calculated from several sources and are displayed to give *approximate* relative values.

Getting Into it

1. A program should begin and progress gradually, especially if you have not been physically active. Start with sessions below your target range and of shorter duration than the recommended half-hour standard.
2. Don't begin a rigorous program without gradual conditioning, even if you have had a stress test that is normal. It is not healthy for either your heart or other muscles in the body.
3. Stop exercising and call your physician if you feel: a) pain or pressure in the center of the chest, the arm, or the throat; b) a very slow pulse when it had been normal or elevated (from exercise) a few moments before; c) a group or groups of very rapid heart beats; or d) faintness, nausea, or vomiting.
4. To avoid muscle, tendon, and joint injuries, stretch the most active mus-

cles before and after exercise and do strengthening exercises for any opposing muscles not used in your main exercise. (See Chapter 11 and Appendix B).

5. Activity should gradually increase over the first five to six weeks to the point where you are reaching your target zone without undue fatigue or shortness of breath. At that time, the ideal exercise session should consist of: a) a 10-minute warm-up below the target range (to prevent injuries and soreness), which includes stretching; b) 30 minutes exercise in (or working up to) the target range; and c) a 10–15-minute cool-down period that includes your main stretching period, and, if you wish, relaxation. Such a 50-minute session should be held three or four days a week.

6. Listen to your body. Be sensible; keep asking, "Is this sensible?" Be aware of your breathing. It is a good indicator of whether you are pushing too hard. If you can talk clearly (though intermittently and slowly) while exercising, then you are not pushing too hard. If you can't talk, slow down.

Dr. Kenneth Cooper's book, *The New Aerobics* (see Resources), gives very detailed instructions on beginning and maintaining a fitness program for a large number of activities.

Over the Long Go

1. Have fun!
2. Always listen to your body, and try to improve your communication with it.
3. Have modest expectations and you will be pleased. You will probably get better with age anyway.
4. Alternate more strenuous and less strenuous days. You will be better for it in the long run. The easy days have the same effect as fertilizing a field —

things will grow better on the other days.

5. Even after you are in condition, take at least one, preferably two, days off a week.
6. You will have difficult (tird, no energy) days. Don't worry about them. Stop if you tire quickly at any time (even in the middle of a "good" day). The next day you will be ready to go again.
7. If you life more than one form of exercise, do more than one. Just don't overdo.
8. Vary your speed, do hills when you can, run figure eights at sometime during your workout and go backwards for a few hundred yards. All of these things increase muscle balance and flexibility.

I run and swim. To some extent these guidelines for an aerobic program reflect my interest. However, they apply equally to bicycling, aerobic dancing, jazzercize, skipping rope, walking, cross-country skiing, and other types of exercise. Find one or two activities that you like and do them. It's the fun and conditioning that matters, not the specific activity.

Aerobic conditioning, flexibility and muscle balance, and muscle building are all desirable outcomes of a regular exercise program. A given individual may want to emphasize one of these more than others, so the chosen program should be designed to achieve the desired outcomes. The necessary preparations and guidelines for a program of aerobic conditioning have been provided, but improved (sometimes even optimal) aerobic conditioning does not always require a specific program. Thus, I have emphasized how your exercise patterns can be significantly expanded by increasing certain kinds of "routine" activities or substituting alternative modes of everyday behavior. As we move now to the chapters on food and eating, remember that regular exercise stabilizes the appetite, can be an indispensable adjunct to weight control, and often contributes to the self-esteem necessary for eating well and in moderation.

RESOURCES CHAPTER 12

Cooper, K.H. *The New Aerobics.* New York: Bantam Books, 1970. Gives the details of the famous Cooper aerobic point system for a number of different aerobic sports.

Cooper, M. and Cooper K.H., *Aerobics for Women.* New York: Bantam Books, 1973.

Fixx, J.F. *The Complete Book of Running.* New York: Random House, 1977. The runners' bible and deservedly so. Covers the technical aspects of running in good detail. Highly readable and well illustrated.

Kuntzleman, B.A. *The Complete Guide to Aerobic Dancing.* New York: Fawcett Books, 1979.

Squires, B. with Krise, R. *Improving Your Running.* Lexington, MA: The Stephen Greene Press, 1982.

13

Eating Poorly, Eating Well

"If doctors of today will not become the nutritionists of tomorrow, the nutritionists of today will become the doctors of tomorrow."

EDISON

WE are in a renaissance of nutritional awareness. More and more professionals and lay people alike acknowledge that how and what we eat is vital to health. Medical schools are beginning to teach nutrition again and the legitimate purview of the subject is no longer just obesity and vitamin deficiency. Many other relationships between nutrition and health have attained widespread acceptance: high-fat diets increase risk for heart disease; fiber lowers risk of bowel cancer. Many others are subtle and still poorly worked out or not even generally recognized such as the effects of food processing on the nutritional value of most foods and the value of refined sugar. However, the most compelling reason for attending to the qualitative issues of nutrition is that people who do so feel better. It isn't a matter of "taking your medicine" to avoid disease; it's really an issue of enjoyment and energy.

Personal Health Competence includes attention to both the qualitative issues and the quantitative aspects of eating. This chapter discusses the qualitative issues; the next chapter focuses on weight management.

THE CURRENT NUTRITIONAL BEHAVIOR OF MOST AMERICANS AND ITS CONSEQUENCES

For the last 50 years Americans have eaten a diet high in fat (average 42 per-

134

cent of total calories), particularly saturated fats (the harder fats like lard, butter, and meat fat, in contrast to oils which are unsaturated), and cholesterol.

Our diet has also been high in refined sugar — 18 percent of calories on the average. In 1976 each American consumed 126 pounds of refined and processed sugar in contrast with less than 40 pounds in 1825 (see Chapter 14). We consume more salt than we need as well. An adult requires less than one-tenth teaspoon per day, but Americans average one to four teaspoons a day. Typical food also contains too little fiber, which is the indigestible part of many vegetables and grains that helps food residues move through the bowel more rapidly. Finally, a significant number of people get more than 10 percent of their total calories from alcohol, which, in addition to its addicting properties, is, like sugar, empty calories.

Table 13-1 summarizes the better known consequences of such poor nutrition, not including vitamin deficiencies. The starred items are discussed in the paragraphs that follow.

Hypertension — High Blood Pressure

There is an important relationship between the intake of salt (sodium chloride) and blood pressure. It is the sodium in salt, as well as other compounds, that is responsible for this relationship. While individuals react differently to high salt intake, the frequency of high blood pressure is related to the level of salt intake in most societies. In the United States, almost every processed food label reveals salt in the enclosed product. Salt is added to baby food to make it taste okay to mothers. Babies don't need it, but it's there, so another salt addict is born. Many people who develop high blood pressure add large amounts of salt to their food, though there are also people who ingest a lot of salt and never get high blood pressure. Some individuals with mild hypertension (blood pressure levels of 140–160/90–105) show significant lowering of blood pressure on restricted sodium intake, although by no means all do. All people who have high blood pressure or who are at some added risk for developing high blood pressure, such as a family history of the condition, are wise to limit their sodium intake. Effectively this means no use of salt at the table, no cooking with salt, and giving up salty processed foods such as potato chips, tortilla chips, pretzels, and pickles.

Recent investigations indicate that a high calcium intake is beneficial for high

TABLE 13–1   The Medical Consequences of Unhealthy Nutrition.

Poor Nutritional Behavior	*Medical Consequence*
too much salt	increased blood pressure* in susceptible people
too much refined sugar	increases weight, empty calories, displaces nutritional food, dental cavities, addiction
too much total and saturated fat, too much cholesterol	increases risk for heart disease*
too many calories (overweight)	increases risk for diabetes, arthritis, high blood pressure, gall bladder disease
too much alcohol	empty calories, liver disease, alcohol addiction, alcoholism, increases risk for some cancers*
too much fat	increases risks for cancer: breast,* colon,* rectum*
low fiber	diverticulitis, bowel cancer, higher blood cholesterol, constipation

blood pressure. When calcium supplements are used, rigid salt restriction is not desirable though excessive use of salt is still harmful.

Coronary Artery Disease

Heart attack and related problems are the leading cause of death in the United States. Volumes of evidence from population studies, laboratory experiments, and clinical observations tell us that there is a definite relationship between the blood (serum) cholesterol level and the chance of developing heart attack. An attack is usually caused by closure of an artery that supplies blood to the heart itself and is due to arteriosclerosis. Some of the same studies, as well as careful experiments in humans involving manipulation of dietary components, show that, for most people, lowering the total fat in the diet will lower the serum cholesterol. In addition there are high correlations between total dietary fat intake in populations (particularly hard fats) and the incidence of coronary disease. People who have high cholesterol or blood sugar need to worry more about their fat intake than those who don't. The intake of vitamins E and B6 and lecithin may also be crucial to preventing arteriosclerosis, though research is still in progress.

Cancer of the Large Bowel and Rectum

A relationship between the amount of fiber in the diet and the incidence of bowel cancer (the more food fiber the less cancer) is increasingly apparent. The time required for food residues to travel from stomach to rectum is the crucial factor. Fiber provides bulk and speeds this process. Because of refined foods and high-fat high refined-sugar intake, the fiber content of the average American diet is very low. Milling flour, for example, removes most of the covering of the wheat kernel, which is the part containing the bran. Bran is largely fiber. Natural foods,

particularly oatmeal and granola, and bread made from whole grain flours are rich in bran. Pure wheat bran sold in natural food stores is inexpensive and, unlike Kellogg's All Bran and some similar products, is whole bran. It tastes like sawdust alone, but is tolerable when mixed with salads or cereals. Corn bran is said to be more effective but is not so readily available.

The frequency of large bowel and rectal cancer is also increased by high alcohol and dietary fat intake over a number of years. High alcohol intake also causes increased incidence of cancers of the lip, mouth, pharynx, esophagus, and stomach. Consumption of more than eight to ten alcoholic beverages a week may be the critical amount, although this is not certain.

Cancer of the Breast

While many factors formerly thought to increase risk for cancer of the breast have been excluded (e.g., being Jewish, never having married, menstruation beginning before 12, daily consumption of alcohol), it now appears that a high fat diet is the most critical risk factor yet identified. Some say the evidence is as compelling as that linking smoking with lung cancer.

HEALTH COMPETENCE IN NUTRITION

To be health competent nutritionally means applying certain basic principles to your eating and gradually changing to an alternative food pattern, the food pattern of health competence.

The Principles of Healthy Eating

The following principles of healthy eating are a synthesis of the current thinking of nutritionists, medical people working in nutrition, and health maintenance enthusiasts. They also incorporate the dietary goals of the Senate Select Subcommittee on Nutrition (1979).

1. *Strive for variety* because a) no single food group contains all the nutrients you need, and b) eating different foods will decrease likelihood of exposure to harmful contaminants that might be found in any one food. Select foods from each of the following groups: a) fresh fruits and vegetables; b) whole grain breads, cereals, other grain products (corn, wheat, rye, rice), c) dry peas, beans (legumes) and nuts; d) animal products—red meat, poultry, fish, milk, yogurt, cheeses. The amounts eaten from group d must be limited. An eight-ounce steak contains 33 grams or 300 calories of saturated fat. This is half the fat intake the average person should have in a day. Also meats are more likely to contain drugs and toxins because the animals are fed grains and often "doctored" with hormones to increase meat production.

2. *Use unprocessed foods* and (in general) non-fat foods—they have more vitamins and minerals per ounce or cupful. Processing can (and usually does) remove, reduce, alter, or destroy these nutrients. It may also add undesirable contaminants. In addition, most processed foods contain a lot of the salt, saturated fat, and sugar that are so prevalent in our diet.

3. *Practice moderation.* It is okay to eat almost anything once in a while but moderation in total calories, salt, fat, cholesterol, sugar, alcohol, and caffeine is healthy.

4. *In certain physiological, stressful, and illness states, compensation is necessary.* Women in the childbearing years may need iron supplements to replace iron lost with menstrual bleeding; pregnant or breastfeeding women need more iron, folic acid, vitamin A, calcium, and calories but most of these can be obtained by properly adjusting the diet. Infants and young children need more vitamins and minerals be-

cause they are growing. Elderly or very inactive people usually eat less, so they should particularly avoid foods high in calories and low in vitamins and minerals like fats, oils, alcohol, and sugars. Persons under inordinate stress and persons with physical or mental ailments need more protein and more calories.

The Alternative Food Pattern

This pattern, the food pattern of health competence, is much more compatible with health and well-being than the typical contemporary American diet. It depends heavily on the first three principles of good nutrition just outlined and helps people to avoid the disorders described previously. In addition, people who have made the change consistently *feel better*, have more energy, and enjoy their food more.

The alternative pattern means more variety (principle 1), fewer processed foods (principle 2), and everything in moderation (principle 3). As a result of these changes, total fat intake decreases, cholesterol intake decreases, salt and refined sugar intake decrease, and the overall caloric density of the food gradually declines. As shown in Table 13-2, you shift from foods predominantly above the line to ones mainly below the line. This involves eating less red meat, fewer high-fat dairy products (butter, cheese), less high cholesterol food, and fewer processed foods (including most fast foods). These are replaced by more whole grains, legumes (mainly beans and peas), fresh fruits and vegetables, and low-fat dairy products—almost all natural foods. It also means replacing foods predominantly on the left side of the table with foods more and more to the right, that is, foods of lower and lower caloric density (less fat and sugar), and less and less processed (more vitamins and minerals, less salt, fat and sugar).

TABLE 13–2 Comparing Prevalent and Alternative Food Patterns[1] [caloric density and salt (Sa), sugar (Su), saturated fat (SF), and cholesterol (C), content of common foods]

Usual U.S. Food Pattern

High Caloric Density (HCD)	*Medium Caloric Density (MCD)*	*Low Caloric Density (LCD)*
Commercial baked goods and cakes made from mixes (SF, C, Sa, Su)	Buttermilk (SF, C, Sa)	Bouillon (Sa)
Frankfurter (SF, C, Sa)	Egg Yolk (SF, C)	Consommé (Sa)
Bacon (SF, C, Sa)	Whole milk (SF, C)	Canned vegetable juice (Sa)
Luncheon meat (SF, C, Sa)	Granolas with added salt and sugar (Sa, Su)	Most canned garden vegetables (Sa)
Ham, sausage (SF, C, Sa)	Shellfish (C)	A few frozen vegetables (peas, succotash, lima beans) (Sa)
Most regular cheeses (SF, C, Sa)	Turkey franks (Sa)	Pickles (Sa)
Ice cream, ice milk (SF, C, Su)	Roasting turkey injected with salt (Sa)	Sauerkraut (Sa)
Creamy peanut butter (SF, Sa)	Canned soups (Sa)	Melba toast (Sa)
Red meat (SF, C)	Canned corn, beans, or peas (Sa)	Salted popcorn (Sa)
Organ meat (SF, C)	Frozen fish (Sa)	
Butter (SF, C)	Canned tuna (Sa)	
Snack crackers (SF, Sa)	Biscuits, muffins, pancakes (Sa)	
Palm oil, coconut oil (SF)	Instant cereals (Sa)	
Hardened margarines (SF)	Dehydrated potatoes (Sa)	
Candy (Su)	All-Bran, Bran flakes, Corn-flakes (Sa)	
Fruit in heavy syrup (Su)	Soda crackers (Sa)	
Sherbet and frozen yogurt (Su)	Soft drinks (Su)	
Salted nuts (Sa)		
Potato chips and other chips (Sa)	*Low in fiber, but otherwise "heart healthy"*	
	White bread, English muffins	
	White rice	
	Spaghetti and other pasta made from white flour	
	Fruit juice without pulp	

Alternative Food Pattern

All vegetable oils *(including olive oil)* except palm and coconut	Breads, lightly milled or whole-grain	Alfalfa sprouts and bean sprouts
Avocado	Brown rice	Artichokes
Honey	Canned fruit (no syrup)	Beets
Mayonnaise or salad dressing	Chicken without skin	Broccoli
Natural peanut butter (no salt)	Common potato and corn	Brussel sprouts
Sesame Butter	Egg whites	Cabbage
Sesame seeds	Fresh fish	Carrots
Soft margarine	Fresh or dried fruit	Cauliflower
Sunflower seeds	Fruit juice with pulp	Celery
Unsalted nuts	Granolas without salt or sugar	Chard
	Legumes (beans, lentils, peas, soy beans, garbanzo beans)	Cucumbers
	Low-fat cottage cheese	Fresh vegetable juice
	Nonfat milk	Green beans
	Puffed rice	Lettuce
	Shredded wheat	Mushrooms
	Spaghetti and other pasta (from partial whole-wheat varieties)	Radishes
	Turkey	Spinach and other greens
	Yams and sweet potatoes	Squash
		Tomatoes and most other garden vegetables
		Most frozen vegetables

1. From Farquhar, John W. *The American Way of Life Need Not Be Hazardous to Your Health* (New York: Norton, 1979). The author is indebted to John W. Farquhar and the Norton Publishing Company, N.Y., N.Y. for permission to reproduce this table.

It is not necessary or even desirable to get entirely below the line or entirely to the right, and it is definitely not necessary to make these changes all at once. In actual practice, it is far better to move into the alternative pattern in several phases, each three to six months long. Each phase can involve relatively easy changes but the *cumulative* effect over two years is a striking alteration in dieting pattern. John Farquhar's book, *The American Way of Life Need Not be Hazardous to Your Health* describes in detail how this phased change process can be accomplished (see Resources).

ABOUT VITAMINS

In the years I've been working on this book, no single question has confused me more than the one of vitamin pills. Some professional nutritionists say we should use supplements and others say a balanced diet will provide enough vitamins. There are experts in health (both physicians and lay people) lined up on both sides of the question. I am not going to summarize the evidence to both views; I favor supplementation. Here are my reasons.

1. The Recommended Daily Allowances (RDA's) for vitamins are felt by many experts to be too low. Dr. Pauling (a Nobel Prize winner in biochemistry some years ago and more recently the most influential and persistent advocate of the use of Vitamin C to prevent and minimize colds) believes we should call the RDA values the Minimum Daily Allowance (MDA) and then propose a Recommended Daily Intake for each vitamin presented as a range instead of just one figure (see Table 13-3).
2. The requirements for a given vitamin can vary from individual to individual. This is true in the "normal"

state of health. Greater variations occur during psychological stress, illness, surgery, physical inactivity, and with aging.
3. Many people do not, or cannot for economic and social reasons, eat nutritionally sound diets.
4. Many medicines antagonize, block, or neutralize the effects of vitamins, and our knowledge about this is very sketchy.
5. Various environmental hazards may increase our need for certain vitamins: pollution, chemicals in food, herbicides, pesticides.
6. Not enough is known about the effects of additives, heat, and cold during the growing, preserving, transporting, and cooking of food (particularly large-scale cooking) on vitamin activities in the food.
7. Our knowledge about all of these things is only beginning to accumulate and be organized in useful ways.

There are a number of multivitamin preparations available that are inexpensive and provide adequate supplementation for average circumstances. Some of my associates take Vitamin E, Vitamin C, and B-complex separately. If you decide to do the latter, I recommend taking two to five times the minimum daily requirement, not more. Personally I do not believe that megavitamin therapy is beneficial. There is ample evidence that it may be harmful in some circumstances.

READING WHAT YOU NEED

The uncertainties of good nutrition are apparent. To some extent we must rely on our own judgment to decide what is good for us and what is bad, what we should eat today and what tomorrow. Although I am not aware of scientific evidence in man to support this contention, I believe we are capable of developing

TABLE 13-3 The Common Vitamins.

Fat-Soluble Vitamin	Main Sources	Properties	Function	Recommended Daily Allowance
A	Cheese, green and yellow vegetables, butter, eggs, milk, fish-liver oils.	Lost by long cooking in open kettle. Toxic in large doses.	Growth, normal bone development, tooth structure, night vision, healthy skin.	4000–5000 IU[b], adults. 2000–3300 IU, child.
D	Fatty fish, eggs, liver, made by skin on exposure to sunlight.	Very stable. Toxic in large doses.	Intestinal absorption of calcium, metabolism of calcium and phosphorous, bone and tooth development.	400 IU.
E	Widely distributed in foods, particularly vegetable oils, wheat germ.	Lost by long cooking in open kettle. Toxic in large doses.	Not definitely known for humans.	30 IU, adult. 20 IU, child.
K	Eggs, liver, cabbage, spinach, tomatoes. Made by intestinal bacteria.	Destroyed by light and alkali. Absorption depends on normal fat absorption.	Blood clotting.	Not established. Given to pregnant women and newborn infants.
Water-Soluble Vitamin				
Thiamin (B₁)	Meat, whole grain, liver, yeast, nuts, eggs, bran, soybeans, potatoes.	Stable in cooking but may dissolve in cooking water. Needed daily.	Carbohydrate metabolism. Promotes growth.	1.0–1.5 mg[d] adult. 0.7–1.2 mg, child.

Vitamin	Sources	Stability	Function	RDA
Riboflavin (B₂)	Milk, cheese, liver, beef, eggs, fish.	Stable in cooking of acid foods Unstable to light and alkali.	Metabolism in all cells.	1.1–1.8 mg, adult. 0.8–1.2 mg, child.
Niacin (nicotinic acid)	Bran, eggs, yeast, liver, kidney, fish, whole wheat, potatoes, tomatoes.	Stable in cooking, may dissolve in cooking water.	Growth, metabolism, normal skin.	12–20 mg, adult. 9–16 mg, child.
B₆ (pyridoxine)	Meat, liver, yeast, whole grains, fish, vegetables.	Stable except to light.	Amino acid metabolism.	1.6–2.0 mg, adult. 0.6–1.2 mg, child.
Folic Acid	Liver, green vegetables.	Not stored; need daily; water soluble.	Division of cells DNA & RNA metabolism.	.4 mg.
B₁₂	Meat, liver, eggs, milk, yeast.	Unstable to acid, alkali, light.	Red blood cells production and growth.	1.0–2.0 ug, adult. 3.0 ug, child.
Ascorbic acid (C)	Citrus fruits, cabbage, tomatoes, potatoes, leafy vegetables.	Very unstable to heat, alkali, air. Dissolves in cooking water.	Cellular metabolism; necessary for teeth, gums, bones, blood vessels.	45 mg, adult. 40 mg, child.

a. Other water-soluble vitamins seem essential to nutrition but are not as well understood, and deficiency is less common.
b. International Units.
c. Retinol Equivalents.
d. Milligrams.
e. Micrograms.
f. Pregnancy and Lactation require 1.5–2.0 times the RDA.

and sharpening a *felt sense* about food — an ability to read our needs. Simply, this means that our bodies will tell us what and how much we need. Yearnings for a particular food are highly significant. If I want dried apricots and nothing else will do, my body is telling me there is something in dried apricots that it is important for me to have. No longer a regular meat eater, I have widely spaced yearnings for red meat. I accede to them. This also happens with certain nuts, a particular fresh vegetable, or fruit. If I keep my diet varied and fresh, I notice these specific yearnings occurring less frequently. Other people with similar food consciousness all say quite definitely that this is a different awareness than their food addictions (usually to sugar or chocolate, which contain no nutrients). I think a tuned mind-body is necessary to activate this sense in a highly refined way. People who are actively exercising and participating in activities that regularly enrich their emotional-spiritual health are more likely to have this sense. In this time of nutritional uncertainty, it is a helpful, perhaps even highly protective mechanism.

THE DEPLETION AND ALTERATION OF FOOD

In the next decade, depletion and alteration of food will be a major controversy in the health field. The following items will provide some appreciation of the magnitude of the problem.

- Most food is grown in depleted soil artificially enriched by chemicals. Changes can occur in the levels of vitamins and protein in grains and other foods as the result of growth assisted by artificial fertilizers.
- Meat and poultry are produced with the aid of hormones and antibiotics. These medicines are used in high enough concentrations so that some of the native material or its metabolic products persist in the meat throughout butchering and processing. They are consumed by the meat eater.
- There is widespread use of insecticides, pesticides, and herbicides in agribusiness. Less well known is the fact that small amounts of these materials are often found in consumer-ready food products. Some are poisons, but their effects on man have not always been adequately studied.
- There are several thousand different (estimates vary from 3–12,000) chemical compounds and additives that may be used to alter or maintain the color, taste, and texture of food, to fortify food that has been depleted during processing, and to prevent premature spoilage. Some single artificial flavorings contain 100 or more untested chemicals. Our ability to monitor additives for safety has not kept pace. Relatively few of them have been tested for safety by the food industry or the FDA. Most people presume food additives are monitored *before they are used.* To emphasize the fallacy of this assumption, Dr. Herbert L. Ley, Jr., former FDA commissioner, said:

  The thing that bugs me is that the people think the FDA is protecting them — it isn't. What the FDA is doing and what the public thinks it is doing are as different as night and day.[2]

- High-volume cooking, freezing, and thawing are commonplace in the preparation of processed foods. Potentially these procedures can deplete food of vitamins and minerals or cause other chemical alterations. There is definite evidence that this is so for some foods, but in the vast majority of instances *we do not know the consequences.*
- The love of Americans for salt and sugar begins with baby food to which

2. *N.Y. Times,* December 31, 1969.

needless salt and sugar are added.

- Although 35 percent of asthmatics are allergic to tartrazine (Yellow #5), it is found as a coloring agent in many anti-asthmatic medications.
- The red dye in one cherry soda can cause cancer in chick embryos.

Recently, the Environmental Protection Agency (EPA) has put severe restrictions on the use of Ethylene Dibromide (EDB) as a pesticide in agriculture. It has been used many years particularly for corn, wheat, and other grains. Before its use, muffin mixes and flour grew weevils after being kept in the home for a while. The government is also going to require that some stored crops be destroyed. For a decade, EDB has been identified as a potent cancer-causing agent in animals. As yet no definite links with human cancer have been shown. But the EPA in its statement says, "It is not acute effects we are concerned about. It is the long-term repeated exposure that may be dangerous." This is 1983. EDB has been used since 1948!

Thus it is obvious that with respect to the qualitative aspects of food, the number of variables is increasing at an enormous rate. Current knowledge is imperfect. We are in an age of nutritional approximation. Most foods are processed. Even fresh fruits and vegetables may be dyed, and most have been grown with pesticides. The situation is complicated by the politics and economics of the food industry. As often occurs under such circumstances, experts, personal experience enthusiasts, and quacks all offer guidance and solutions. Even those programs which are sound involve principles counter to established eating habits and, often, economic capability.

There are no easy answers for consumers about how to deal with these problems. Packaging laws do not require that all additives be mentioned on the label, so it behooves all of us to keep informed as well as possible, to express concern when we feel it, and to boycott any products for which there is good evidence of harmful effects. Eating a variety of foods and unprocessed foods as often as possible will minimize the unknown dangers, but unfortunately, under present controls, not make us immune to serious harm.

In these pages, we reviewed the prevalent pattern of eating in the U.S. and its harmful consequences. A contrasting food pattern that minimizes those harmful outcomes and is based on sound nutritional principles was presented. My own conclusions about vitamin supplementation and words of caution about the potential poisons in our food were discussed. In the next chapter the health competence of weight management will be outlined. As you read it, remember that the qualitative aspects of nutritional health competence are doubly important if a person is controlling or losing weight. They are an integral part of any program of weight control.

RESOURCES CHAPTER 13

Ballentine, R. *Diet and Nutrition.* Hinesdale, PA: Himalayan International Institute, 1978. A comprehensive and authoritative analysis of many of the most crucial aspects of nutrition.

Farquhar, J. *The American Way of Life Need Not be Hazardous to Your Health* (see General Resources).

Hall, R.H. *Food for Nought, The Decline in Nutrition.* New York: Harper and Row, 1974. A critical analysis of the current qualitative issues in nutrition. Comprehensive and provocative. The author is a prestigious biochemist.

14

Body Fat and Weight Management

Weight loss must be the by-product of personal evolution. The person who tackles the weight problem head-on, as though *it* is the basic issue, is doomed to fail. If one does not truly outgrow being fat, he will lose (and gain) tons in a long and unhappy career of dieting struggles.[1]

OVERWEIGHT people are more likely to develop high blood pressure, diabetes, back problems, certain kinds of arthritis, and gall bladder disease. Due to reduced dexterity and quickness, some heavy people are more prone to accidents. The culturally induced adverse effects of obesity on self-esteem and employability are considerable. The magnitude of the problem is large. It is estimated that 30 percent of all Americans are significantly "overweight." The *average* person in the United States is 20 pounds "overweight." Thus, weight management is definitely an important skill in health competence.

Weight control is a common problem because it is a difficult one. We have to eat. Unlike tobacco and mood-altering substances, we must have food. In addition, overeating and snacking are clearly tied to emotional factors and long-ingrained habits; food often compensates for other unmet needs. The cultural pressure in our society to be thin is immense and greatly complicates rational approaches to weight management. The diet industry is essentially self-perpetuating, not, as might be expected, putting itself out of business. For these reasons, *weight control involves changing the way we live with food.* Most over-

1. R. Ballentine, *Diet and Nutrition* (Hinesdale, PA: Himalayan International Institute, 1978).

144

weight people lose a lot of weight during their lives. It is unchanged behaviors that put it back on again. Obesity is truly an illness, not a disease. It has both underlying psychological causes and creates its own psychological problems.

SUZANNE'S STORY

Suzanne is a 42-year old professional woman, married, with three children. She has "always been overweight, at least from 9 or 10 on." Two episodes from adolescence are particularly vivid. The first occurred when she visited a carnival at age 13. There she won a prize when the inevitable "If I don't guess your weight within three pounds, you get a prize" person estimated her weight 12 pounds too low. The second episode was much more aversive. Once, at least, her father measured her thighs and compared them with his own, which were smaller. He jeered at her.

Until recently, Suzanne's father would greet her on the phone by saying, "Hi, Fatty." When she finally asked him to stop he did, but still insists that she is being oversensitive. Recently, an aunt whom she had not seen for many years, told her she was "too fat." Messages from her husband are, on the one hand, that he doesn't mind her being fat, but on the other, "I want you to lose weight for your health."

Suzanne has enjoyed pregnancy because it "gave me an excuse to look fat." She nursed her infants and gained weight or maintained some of the added pregnancy weight each time. "I couldn't diet when nursing." This difficulty seemed to have a physical component, "Always hungry, ate constantly," and an emotional one, "When nursing, I felt like a mother," and there's a difference between a mother ("for whom it doesn't matter if you're fat") and a woman ("women should be thin").

Suzanne emphasized that until having children in the last five years she didn't "try very hard" to lose weight. "I knew I should, but I just felt chunky." The hard thing about dieting used to be that when "you go off it you feel awful (about yourself), like a failure." This was inevitably followed by "what's the use" feelings, "and then you just fall off the diet." Psychotherapy has now improved

her confidence and self-esteem to the point where she now accepts her flaws and so, "it's much easier to stay on a diet. It isn't such a big deal when you mess up for a day or so; you can go back on, and it's okay."

After her third child, she gained weight while nursing. She then dieted earnestly for the first time and sought a doctor's advice. He gave her a 1200-calorie diet and made further support optional. He didn't describe the support plans available, recommend exercise, or help Suzanne clarify the benefits for her of overeating.

Suzanne said that after 20 pounds of weight loss she had now been stable five months. She felt anxious because people were telling her how good she looked and how great it was that she was losing weight. She feared she might have cancer. Then she said, "I think I have some resistance to being really thin . . . Everything I've told you so far hasn't been particularly difficult, but I don't want to tell you how much I weigh."

I asked her to elaborate on her resistance. "I feel like I would be a different person . . . somehow I associate being thin with a racy, sexually aggressive, and promiscuous life style, and that scares me a lot. It would also make me feel more vulnerable . . . Nobody will rape me the way I am but if I got thin they might."

This story illustrates a number of important points:

1. The unhelpful messages that overweight people can get from their "loved" ones.
2. How unhelpful physicians can be for someone who wants (or needs) to lose weight. The story of being handed (or told) a diet without other help is not an unusual one.
3. The important relationship between self-image and readiness to initiate serious change. Suzanne "didn't try very hard" until after therapy had significantly increased her self-esteem. Certainly her most dramatic weight gain also increased her motivation, but new-found comfort with her own

imperfections decreased the likelihood that she would give up because of a brief slip.

4. How complex and profound the perceived and unperceived benefits of fatness can be. In Suzanne's instance, the major benefit was protection from two frightening spectors: potential involvement in more varied and experimental sexual encounters, and increased vulnerability.

WHAT IS OVERWEIGHT? INTRODUCING PERCENT BODY FAT

Until recently, overweight was generally defined as a 10 percent or greater increase over ideal weight, as defined by standard tables (Table 14-1). The ideal weight table reflects recent upward revision (5–10 percent) by the life insurance companies. Claims are being made that the new values are not valid because they

TABLE 14–1   Standard Weight Table.

Men

Height	Small	Medium	Large
5'2"	128–134	131–141	138–150
5'3"	130–136	133–143	140–153
5'4"	132–138	135–145	142–156
5'5"	134–140	137–148	144–160
5'6"	136–142	139–151	146–164
5'7"	138–145	142–154	149–168
5'8"	140–148	145–157	152–172
5'9"	142–151	148–160	155–176
5'10"	144–154	151–163	158–180
5'11"	146–157	154–166	161–184
6'0"	149–160	157–170	164–188
6'1"	152–164	160–174	168–192
6'2"	155–168	164–178	172–197
6'3"	158–172	167–182	176–202
6'4"	162–176	171–187	181–207

Women

Height	Small	Medium	Large
4'10"	102–111	109–121	118–131
4'11"	103–113	111–123	120–134
5'0"	104–115	113–125	122–137
5'1"	106–118	115–129	125–140
5'2"	108–121	118–132	128–143
5'3"	111–124	121–135	131–147
5'4"	114–127	124–138	134–151
5'5"	117–130	127–141	137–155
5'6"	120–133	130–144	140–159
5'7"	123–136	133–147	143–163
5'8"	126–139	136–150	146–167
5'9"	129–142	139–153	149–170
5'10"	132–145	142–156	152–173
5'11"	135–148	145–159	155–176
6'0"	138–151	148–162	158–179

These tables were published in 1983 by the Metropolitan Life Insurance Company. All weights are with shoes; men's weight include 5 and women's include 3 pounds of indoor clothing.

were not corrected for smoking. Smokers weigh less than most people the same height and weight, and in calculating the ideal weights, the mortality for a given weight was apparently not corrected for smoking.

Today it is considered more meaningful to measure percentage of body fat, rather than rely solely on such charts. This can be done easily with skin fold calipers and an equation or tables, but immersion tank methods are more accurate. How do you know if you are over-fat? Various percent values are shown in the following table. The average values do not reflect optimal levels of fat.

The "recommended values" are shown together with the values used to define obesity. For comparison the average values in young adults are shown as well as those in elite runners. In later adult life the average U.S. values rise rapidly and far exceed the recommended values shown in Table 14-2. Body fat measurements are most useful in muscular, apparently overweight people. In those who are relatively inactive, excess weight measured on a scale will accurately reflect increases in body fat.

TABLE 14-2 Body Fat as Percentage of Total Body Weight.

Recommended Values (General Population)	
Women	25% or less
Men	20% or less
Average Values in Young Adults	
Women	26%
Men	15%
Values in Elite Runners	
Women	8–11%
Men	6–8 %

BASIC FACTORS THAT CONTROL WEIGHT

Caloric Balance

Weight is stable when caloric expenditure is equal to caloric intake. Calories expended increase (providing fat to muscle ratios remain the same) with a person's size and invariably with increased activity. The caloric expenditure of a few different activities is shown in Table 12-2. No one will lose fatty tissue weight (as opposed to fluid weight) without reducing caloric intake below caloric needs.

Appetite Set Point

Each of us apparently has a narrow range of normal appetite, a "set point" which is resistant to change. However, it is lowered by smoking (nicotine), some appetite reducing drugs (the amphetamines), and exercise. If a previous inactive person does vigorous exercise on a regular basis, the set point will decrease as the person loses weight (if they were overweight to start with). Any one individual may not continue to shed weight all the way to their ideal level without further increases in exercise (depending upon how much exercise they were doing in the first place). This "set point theory" has given some comfort to overweight people, but the critical question must be whether the set point found when people are studied in the overweight state is the same as they had before becoming overweight.

Appetite in Relation to Particular Foods

Recent work suggests what many dieters have insisted all along, that the kind of food a person eats affects appetite and, therefore, chances of losing weight. In a general way, foods high in table or refined sugar increase appetite within the next few hours. Fruit sugar, by contrast (as well as many other foods), generally doesn't increase appetite. The effects of any food on appetite (see Table 14-3) are apparently related to the degree to which they stimulate the secretion and raise blood levels of insulin. The blood insulin level appears to have more to do with appetite control than the level of blood sugar. When food containing glucose or sucrose is eaten, blood sugar rises rapidly followed closely by a rise in insulin levels. The insulin then stays elevated two to three hours. Fruit sugar (and many other foods) causes a slower rise in blood sugar and a slower, lower rise in blood insulin levels. Table sugar contains both glucose and fructose (fruit sugar), but acts in this regard like pure glucose.

In Table 14-3 some common foods are separated into low-range, medium-range, and high-range groups depending on their ability to stimulate rises in blood insulin level. Most of the low range insulin stimulators (non-appetite stimulators) contain some fat or protein in addition to carbohydrate. So apparently these substances can mask or subdue the insulin stimulating effect of sugar (glucose). Ice cream, one of the country's favorite sweets, is such an example.

pens because fatty tissue infiltrates muscle tissue. Often activity slows because of increased body mass. As the percentage of body fat rises, the basic energy needs of the body decline (at least in proportion to total weight) so that the heavier someone gets, the harder it is to lose weight.

A corollary of this is that dieting without an exercise program (a program of increased activity) is foolhardy. When weight is lost without exercising, about half of what is lost is muscle. When the weight is regained (after most crash diets), all of what is gained back is fat. So the person is worse off than when he or she started, even though the weight returns to the same level.

OTHER FACTS ABOUT WEIGHT CONTROL

The successful reduction of weight and body fat is based on attention to both of

TABLE 14–3 Insulin Stimulating Potential of Foods and Sugars*.

Low Range	Medium Range	High Range
fructose	sucrose	glucose
skim milk	white spaghetti	honey
whole milk	bananas	corn flakes
ice cream	raisins	carrots
yoghurt	frozen peas	parsnips
dried beans and peas	pastry	rice
lima beans	whole wheat spaghetti	wheat and white bread
peanuts	oatmeal	shredded wheat
sausages	all bran	beets
fish sticks	apples	white potatoes
tomato soup	oranges and orange juice	Mars bar
	sweet potatoes and yams	
	baked beans	

*The table and some of the written material is adapted from *Taming the Hunger Hormone* by Judith Rodin, PhD., *American Health*, Jan/Feb 1984, p. 43.

Altered Metabolism in Fat People

As a person gets more and more overweight, their percentage of body fat rises. As this occurs, the proportion of muscle tissue, which burns far more energy, to fatty tissue increases. Initially this hap-

the following principles: first, that people become overweight because they consume more calories than they burn; second, problems of overweight and obesity are based on complex interrelationships between mind and body (see Figure 14-1).

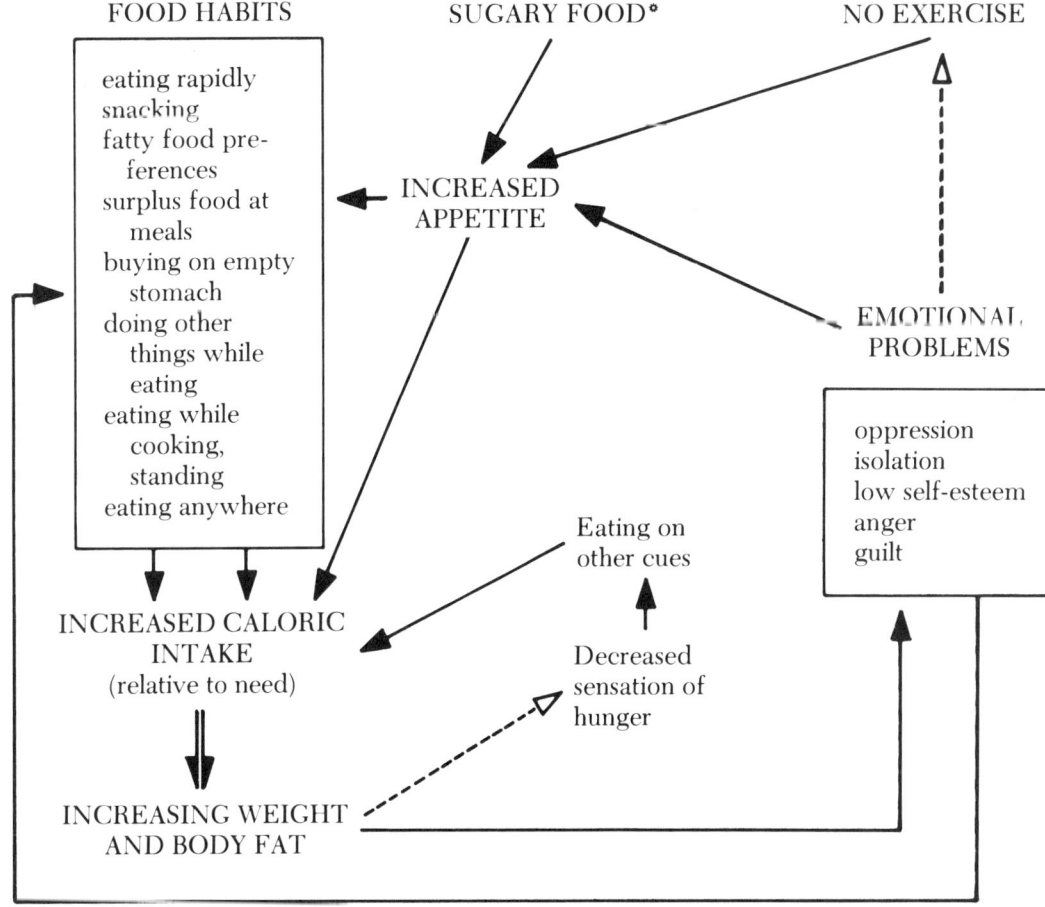

°"SUGARY FOOD" = food high in sucrose or dextrose

FIGURE 14–1   Behavioral and Physiological Factors in Eating.

The following facts are basic. They will save a lot of disappointment. There is no "easy" way to lose weight.

1. It requires a deficit of 3,500 calories (that is, a person must burn 3,500 more calories than they consume) in order to lose one pound. A person must walk or run 35 miles to burn 3,500 calories.

2. To the basic caloric requirement, one must add any additional calories required by physical activity. To lose weight, caloric intake must be less than the total of the basic requirement and the additional requirement of physical activity.

3. For overweight but otherwise normal people not taking medications, *weight can vary as much as three pounds in a 24-hour period*, if measured on arising or more if measured at different times of the day. For most people this variation is less, but for people with high blood pressure or heart disease who are taking medications, it can be even more. *Don't be discouraged or overly encouraged by day-to-day weight differences. In fact, don't rely on them.*

4. On almost any diet, the initial weight loss is largely fluid, not loss of fatty tissue. In the first three or four days on a low-calorie diet (one that is 500

or more calories below requirements), it is possible to lose three to five pounds in fluid, sometimes more. The "immediate" results of many "miracle" diets are based on nutritional manipulations. Fluid loss increases early in the diet and provides apparent instant success. Conversely, a high-carbohydrate intake that begins after a period of negative caloric balance can result in the re-accumulation of fluid and a three-to-four pound weight gain in 24 hours.

5. For most people near normal weight who go without food for some time, reductions in blood sugar and contractions of the stomach stimulate hunger. These occur in overweight people, too, but some do not perceive them. Their hunger responds instead to external signals: the presence of food, emotional upset, other kinds of stress. Some say, for example, that fear, which causes reduction in appetite for most people of normal weight, can cause an increase in food intake in the obese.

SOME GUIDELINES THAT ARE HELPFUL IN LOSING WEIGHT

1. Increase physical activity. This will prevent loss of muscle tissue as well as burn calories. Begin an exercise program when you begin weight reduction. Make it something that's easy to do. Walking is best for most people because it just requires allowing more time to get places. Walking briskly 30 minutes a day will use up 180 calories; walking an hour will use 360. The best time is just before the evening meal, since exercise will also reduce appetite. See the preceding chapter for suggestions on increasing your exercise as part of everyday living. Once you are walking briskly two or more miles a day,

a more vigorous aerobic program can be gradually adopted.

2. Mobilize a support system. Use contracts or letters to people you eat with asking them to encourage (not subvert) your efforts.

3. Do your program with a group of other weight losers if possible. Meet with them regularly; I recommend Overeaters Anonymous. Compare experience, notes, difficulties, and emotional reactions.

4. Gradually modify your diet to decrease high-caloric density foods like fatty foods, sugar foods, alcohol, red meat, while increasing medium and low-caloric density foods, and move from processed foods to unprocessed foods. In my experience, people who want to lose weight find a phased and gradual shift to an alternative food pattern much more acceptable and manageable than going cold turkey on rich (by definition, high-caloric density) foods they love.

In following the alternative diet adhere to the dietary principles explained in the previous chapter. They are more important than ever when losing weight. Within the limits, which they establish:

a. Eat three meals a day. Don't skip breakfast.

b. Avoid foods high in sugar or fat, but do include starches such as whole wheat bread, potatoes, or rice.

c. Limit portion size of meat; even lean meat is high in calories.

d. Use non-fat and low-fat dairy products.

e. Eat slowly, making each meal last for 30 minutes without second helpings.

f. Decide on one mid-morning and one mid-afternoon snack if you become hungry between meals.

g. Plan low-calorie snacks ahead of

time. Fruits and vegetables are ideal. Eat slowly, spending at least 10 minutes on each snack.

h. Expect weight loss to be slow but steady. Better to lose 10 pounds a year and keep it off than to lose 10 pounds one month and regain it the next.

i. Don't use diet pills; use laxatives only for constipation.

j. Drastically limit or stop using foods containing a lot of free sugar. They increase your appetite.

5. Throw away all diet books which advocate a simple answer (such as a high-protein diet) or ones that severely restrict calories. They may be bad for your health; they don't supply all the nutrition you need, and they are almost impossible to stick with. They don't work; 90 percent of the people who lose weight on these diets gain it back.

6. Work with a program, group or therapist to change your self-image from that of a fat person to that of a thin person (see Resources, *Diets Don't Work*).

7. Plan on no more than one pound a week weight loss. Two pounds per month is fine. Plan a total program, including stabilization, of one to three years in duration. Phase the longer changes (6-month or 12-month phases) you make in your eating patterns.

8. Don't get down on yourself for "blowing a day." *No one* is perfect, and it's okay. It's only the long-term changes in behavior that will make a lasting difference anyway.

9. Reward yourself for reaching interim goals, but not with food. Buy yourself a present or take a couple of hours off, or whatever. But get in the habit of providing rewards.

10. While dieting, it is wise to take a vitamin supplement. A once-a-day multivitamin preparation is adequate.

11. Weigh yourself only on two consecutive days a week (midweek is best). Always do it in the morning before eating or drinking anything and wear no clothes or the same clothes. Use the same scale in exactly the same place. Record the average of the two days as your weight for the week. This will avoid some of the discrepancies that occur because of fluid variations and variable patterns of retention of food residues in the bowel.

12. Keep a journal for about one week in every three of what you eat, when, and why. Record associated events in your life. This will help you to follow suggestion 13 and learn what your patterns are. In particular it will help you relate certain stressful events to the act of eating.

13. Analyze your behavior. Try to learn what eating does for you. (See Chapter 10.) Whatever the benefits are, they are probably important (provide comfort, combat loneliness, make you less nervous). Therefore, you will have to find another way to gain the same benefits. See how certain eating patterns contribute to your caloric intake and interfere with your progress in losing weight. These include (see Figure 14-1): eating rapidly, snacking, using high-caloric density foods, having surplus food at meals, little exercise, buying on an empty stomach, eating problem foods, eating in numerous places, doing other things while eating, eating while cooking or standing.

WOMEN AND WEIGHT LOSS: OTHER PERSPECTIVES

Among advocates for women's health, there is considerable concern that women are persuaded and intimidated to try and lose weight for the wrong reasons. A number of major industries (clothing, cosmetics, food, dieting) depend for a major proportion of their business on the dollars of women who are persuaded they are unattractive if their body forms do not resemble Farrah Fawcett's or Jane Fonda's. Those concerned feel that the majority of women trying to lose weight are motivated by culturally determined ideals that have little to do with health. Many men validate and strengthen this construct through casual comments, jokes, standards, and frank appraisals.

As a result, women are prone to try weight reduction methods that are not safe, are not likely to have permanent results, and, for a significant number of dieting women, are not necessary for reasons of health in the first place. I am in basic agreement. The motivation for most dieting is culturally determined rather than health determined. The alarming increase in the number of women with anorexia nervosa (compulsive undereating), bulimia (compulsive vomiting), and other eating disorders supports these contentions.

In her book, *Fat is a Feminist Issue*, Susie Orbach has yet another perspective. She makes the case for fat (at least in most women) not being about food, but rather being about protection, sex, mothering, strength, and love. She says it is a response to the way women are seen by the important people in their lives and by themselves. She urges that they view weight management as a good thing, not as a punishment, and helps them learn how to do that. She is taking the whole theory of "benefits" (See Chapter 10) and their importance to people and applying the idea to women and diet.

Finally, a more recent group of authors takes issue with the assumption that being fat is detrimental to health. Their basic argument is that health hazards are a direct result of the tension and stress created by the cultural and political pressures mentioned above. The assumption is that if the cultural pressures were removed that even grossly overweight people would not have higher incidence of gall bladder disease, arthritis, heart attack, or high blood pressure. My own feeling is that this claim is worth our attention, and that as with many controversies of this kind, the truth lies somewhere in between the extreme views. The stress originating from cultural pressures probably does create or worsen some of the disability and problems, but may have little to do with others.

I believe excess body fat and being overweight are, at least in part, health issues. However, what is being said in these various perspectives demands further attention and is worth appropriate investigation.

Weight management is one of the most difficult aspects of health competence. When achieved it serves as a firm basis for increased well-being, self-esteem, and physical capability. The guidelines outlined in this chapter are based on sound nutrition and good principles of emotional-spiritual health. They are also based on the belief that being fat is not healthy. This view is being vigorously challenged by the women's health movement and others. They say that the increase of certain medical problems in overweight people results from the stress attendant upon the political and cultural oppression of fat people. These views represent important concerns and lines of thinking that need to be heard and investigated.

RESOURCES CHAPTER 14

Ballentine. *Diet and Nutrition* (Cited in Chapter 13).

Brand Name Calorie Counter — a number are available in most bookstores. Though I do not advocate counting calories, a book like this is useful in helping you detect the hidden calories in many processed foods and in learning what the high caloric density foods are.

Farquhar, J. *The American Way of Life Need Not be Hazardous to Your Health* (see General Resources).

Orbach, S. *Fat is a Feminist Issue.* New York: Berkeley Books, 1979. Discussed in this chapter.

Overeaters Anonymous. See citation in Chapter 10. OA is patterned after AA and, unlike practically all other weight management programs is not commercial. Like AA there is a lot of emphasis on learning how to live in ways that will diminish the need for compulsive eating.

Schwarz, B. *Diets Don't Work.* Houston: Breakthrough Publishing, 1982.

Weight Watchers. The oldest and best known of the commercial programs. Weight Watchers can be extremely useful for the individual who needs some extrinsic motivation to succeed.

Part V

The Pathway of Illness and Problem Care

> Each patient carries his own doctor inside him. They come to us not knowing the truth. We are at our best when we give the doctor who resides within each patient a chance to go to work.
>
> ALBERT SCHWEIZER[1]

EARLIER I spoke of the American Indian philosophy that illness is a teacher. It is also frequently a friend. Although illness causes pain and suffering, it also challenges us to confront ourselves to be open to changing the course of our lives. If we accept this kind of challenge, illness can bring learning and growth that we might have previously thought impossible.

Repeatedly I see people's lives changed in the most profound ways by illness. They learn more about who and what they are, mobilize inner resources they didn't know existed, or get in touch for the first time with their own spirit or their God. Thus, although illness can be profoundly disquieting, painful, and frustrating, it will always prove instructive in some way if permitted to do so. Illness *is* a teacher. Part of health competence is learning to deal effectively, respectfully, and positively with illness when it comes.

One impediment to positive experience with illness can be difficulty working with the medical care system and physicians. Therefore, much of Part V is devoted to doing a more effective job of working with your physician, not only as a diagnostician and therapist, but as an important advisor, ally, and resource person. Part V begins with a look at the Person-Doctor Relationship, how it works, and a number of the ways in which it is commonly defective. The idea of partnership is introduced, and the beliefs and skills requisite to partnership

1. Jaffe, *Healing from Within* (see Chapter 6 Resources).

laid out. The remaining chapters discuss more specific situations in which the partnership concept and skills can be fruitfully applied.

I hope this part of the book will bring more satisfaction to the person-provider relationship for both parties. Although it focuses on the medical care process from the consumer's perspective, it can also guide health professionals who want to re-examine their role and effectiveness in the person-provider relationship. Since patient is largely an inappropriate term to use when talking about health, self-responsibility, and involvement, I have used person or customer instead. This is admittedly confusing at times — particularly when the term "person-doctor relationship" is used, since doctors are definitely people, too!

15

The Person-Doctor Relationship: Present Reality, Future Hope

PATIENT OR PERSON?

IN this era the word "patient" is often misused. The noun "patient" is: "an individual awaiting or under medical care or treatment; one that is acted upon." The adjective "patient" means: "bearing pains or trials calmly or without complaint; manifesting forbearance under provocation or strain; able or willing to bear."

While the first of the nominal definitions is unobjectionable, the second decribes patient non-responsibility and non-involvement — "one that is acted upon." The adjectival meanings also accurately describe what doctors, other health care personnel, and hospitals usually appear to expect of their customers. Until 25 years ago, most people under medical care were accurately described by terms like "bearing pains or trials calmly or without complaint." Now, however, many seeking "medical" assistance have stable chronic illness, are interested in health maintenance, or simply have questions. When they have a more acute problem they want to be responsible and are not interested in passivity or collusion. Even if they do not want responsibility, they desire dignity.

I prefer the word "person" or "customer" rather than "patient." This will not change the way things work, but it can raise awareness of both physicians and their customers that many individuals do not want a constantly authoritarian relationship. They go to a physician wanting attention for themselves, not only for their disease. These are persons, not patients. We are in a

157

time in which many people who are suffering or anguished from disease or injury also desire fuller participation in their own care—and in that way are persons.

THE PERSON-DOCTOR RELATIONSHIP

For almost everyone a relationship with a physician is at the core of their *personal* medical (but not necessarily health) care system. This person-doctor relationship (which I will call the PDR) is the framework in which medical care is initiated and proceeds. Physicians provide access to care through their offices, the emergency room, and the hospital. They control the frequency of contact, the direction and quality of the diagnostic and therapeutic steps, and the dispensation of education, solace, and caring.

All problems experienced in obtaining good medical care cannot be attributed to physicians, people, or the relationship between them. But in most circumstances the PDR is the key to more effective, self-participative, pleasant care. To be effective, you must know how it works, what can go wrong with it, and how to fix it. More important, you need to learn to prevent or minimize difficulties and problems in the first place.

In the chapter on relationships, I stated that people who have effective, growing relationships acknowledge that nothing that happens in that relationship is the responsibility of only one party. When something goes well or poorly in a person-doctor relationship, the person and the doctor are both responsible. Engaging in an effective relationship with a health provider is part of Personal Health Competence.

Listening to people talk about their experience with doctors is revealing and discouraging. Comments like these are often heard:

"I have to wait so long in the office."

"Doc doesn't treat me like a person, just like a sore foot."

"I feel like I can't talk to him. He's so busy."

"I wonder what pill the doc'll give me for this."

I also listen to physicians talk to and about their patients:

"If you'd taken better care of your leg, this wouldn't have happened."

"My patients never do what I *tell* them."

"People just don't come to see me soon enough; you'd think they'd know better."

Each of these statements is real for the person who made it. The average consumer is dissatisfied with and often antagonistic toward their medical care. In their medical affairs, people lack self-confidence, feel generally inferior and powerless, and make few real choices. Many are indifferent.

Physician's lives and work are not always satisfactory either. The average doctor does make an ample income (some are outrageous) and to all appearances has security and a happy life. Most work very hard, have little personal time, and feel isolated, because it is an ethic in medicine not to show and talk about feelings although medical work arouses powerful ones all the time. People may call and make visits to the office inappropriately, complain disproportionately, be pathologically dependent, and sue without ample justification. Physicians may practice defensive medicine, which means they order many tests and X-rays just to be covered if later sued. Often they do not enjoy their work, "burnout," and keep going anyway.

WHAT'S BEHIND UNSATISFACTORY PERSON-DOCTOR RELATIONSHIPS

Most problems in the person-physician relationship can be traced to four interacting factors: 1) a disparity in "world views"; 2) the problem of collusion; 3) a lack of love and creativity; 4) the expectation of patient compliance.

The Disparity in World Views

Physicians are (or act like they are) mainly interested in disease, not people, and in sickness, not health. People, on the other hand *expect* physicians to be interested in them as whole persons and in their staying well, not just getting better when they are sick.

It is the rare physician who consistently works with the person *and* his or her concerns, who treats disease when it is present, but also views a doctor's work as encompassing the person and *all* legitimate concerns (bodily changes, psychological problems, and practical matters) that are a consequence of the medical problem. Most physicians regard their work as disease and the curing of disease, but not illness and the healing of illness. (See the mind-body connection, Chapter 6.) This is compounded by physicians who persist in ordering more and more tests in hopes that "something" will be found. This is usually for the doctor's comfort, not the patient's. Eventually, the results may suggest a problem, which in turn elicits more "technical" responses from the physician.[1] This is usually a poor alternative to probing the patient's deeper concerns, thereby getting to the *real* problem.

People often expect something quite different. Whether or not they consider the physician's work to be a blend of curing and healing, they expect at some level to be *healed*. By definition this means they must be regarded as whole people, be treated kindly and with compassion, and have the physician recognize both the broad roots and the impact of their sickness.

1. There are times when such a hunt turns up disease. The skillful physician knows when and when not to proceed.

Many people also seek greater self-determination and involvement, attention to health maintenance and well-being, the use of alternatives to drugs and surgery, and greater awareness of the body-mind connection. When these expectations are not met, disappointment, frustration, and dissatisfaction are all inevitable and interfere with the person-physician process.

Collusion

This disparity in world views is magnified by collusion between most person-physician pairs. In the following story, Bud and his doctor pretend that Bud's health is better than it is. The doctor underplays Bud's risks, and Bud who is actually worried about himself, fails to bring them up.

Bud is a 40-year old white-collar worker. He is about 25 pounds overweight; his blood pressure is under 140/90 (at least it usually comes down to that while he sits in the physician's office), and he has no particular pain or other evidence of abnormal body function. His doctor calls him healthy. He does smoke 15 cigarettes a day, routinely has one or two drinks with lunch and three more before dinner, works under pressure most of his 55-hour work week, takes work home, barely manages an hour a week with his children, and has little interest in sex. His doctor, who is disease-oriented, chooses to ignore these multiple risks for heart attack (Bud's electrocardiogram is normal). In a real sense, his doctor regards Bud as no more or less healthy than his counterpart who runs three miles a day, limits working evenings to one a week, works hard at his marital and family relationships, doesn't smoke, maintains normal weight, never has had a blood pressure higher than 125/80, and has a satisfying sex life.

If pressed, the physician does admit that Bud is indeed at greater risk of becoming ill—particularly of succumbing to a heart attack—but he fails to use this knowledge to assess and guide Bud's health program. He gives him a clean bill, mentions that he should have his blood pressure checked again in a few months and "waits." Bud in turn is troubled by his smoking, wonders about his blood pressure, pot belly, and sexual disinterest, but says nothing.

The Lack of Love and Creativity

Still another phenomenon, perhaps the most important one, goes on between doctors and patients. "Doesn't go on" is more accurate. There is not a lot of love moving between people and their physicians. Again, love is defined as a commitment to support another's growth as a person. Too many doctors fix people like mechanics fix cars, so they can go on, basically unchanged except for the new parts or the fixed piece. For their part, people do not support the doctor in growing: in becoming more comfortable at being with people, talking to them, or telling them bad news, physically comforting them, or doing whatever is required to enrich the spirit or soul. So people who come to their physicians with hurt, concern, or dysfunction, which provides an enormous opportunity to grow, lose that opportunity. Similarly, the physician also misses his opportunity to grow.

In the absence of love, the potential for personal growth and creativity on the part of both the physician and the person is not realized. An encounter between physician and person is almost like passing in the night.

The Expectation of Patient Compliance

Although the issue of compliance is, in fact, an outgrowth of the deficiency of love, it is important enough to have its own space. In recent years, patient education has received a wave of attention. Many physicians, nurses, and hospitals are enthusiastic. They sincerely believe that a better job of educating people about what is wrong with them will result in better "patients," and health care

would improve. One characteristic of a "better patient," as defined by these enthusiasts, is that the person does what he or she is told to do more reliably — *the patient is more compliant*. Thus the physician often views the degree of patient compliance as an indicator of how much responsibility the person has assumed for his or her own health. The "noncompliant" person is generally viewed as unwilling to accept responsibility and less likely to have successful outcomes.

Before such a conclusion can be drawn, the tendency to view patient compliance as a desired goal must be challenged. Webster defines compliance as "giving in to a request, wish, demand; a tendency to give in to others; submissive." Given this definition, it is incongruous to assume that compliant people have assumed responsibility for their health. Instead, a compliant patient may resign responsibility for his or her own body, giving that control to the physician. Conversely, the noncompliant patient retains greater self-responsibility and authority, which is not necessarily at the expense of illness-producing behavior.

Some people, when ill, do prefer (sometimes need) to be given orders and follow them carefully, particularly the critically ill. However, the physician who routinely creates such an authoritarian relationship places patients who want to retain some authority within the doctor-patient relationship in the difficult position of noncompliance.

Let's contrast Bud and his physician with Ted and Dr. Field.[2]

Ted is a 52-year-old man who is used to power. Each day, as chief executive of a bank, he makes decisions involving large sums of money, decisions that influence the lives and fortunes of many. He is known in

2. This example was described by Naomi Ruben, M.D., then medical editor of the Institute for the Study of Humanistic Medicine.

his field for his good judgment, his ability to take cooly and confidently the risks necessary for progress.

Ted appeared in Dr. Field's office one morning complaining of a cough and shortness of breath. Typically hurried, he demanded, "What's my problem? Find out and do something. I must be in my office this afternoon." Although Ted was impatient with his questions, Dr. Field persevered and obtained a history suggestive of pneumonia. On examining and listening to Ted's chest, the physician was not surprised to find abnormal sounds that suggested pneumonia on both sides. An X-ray and blood counts confirmed his impression of bacterial pneumonia.

Ted returned to the office and sat down, a powerful but obviously ill man. He was anxious to return to work and seemingly unwilling to allow his body the time it needed to resolve his infection. Field wondered how to enable Ted to use his good judgment to help himself. Speaking with the authority of his doctor status, he could have told him what it was he should do—what amount of rest, what drugs, what tests. But this man, not used to accepting authority, might oppose his own needs if presented to him this way.

So Field put the problem in Ted's hands. He showed him his X-rays and said, "Ted, this density is pneumonia. Your white count suggests that it is bacterial rather than viral. Judging from your story, the infection has been present at least two days. What do you think you should do about this?"

Ted eyed his physician the way he might eye an employee who is not competent. "Well, you are the doctor," he said. "Yes, I know. But what are your thoughts about the situation?" Ted thought briefly then formulated a plan of action. "It looks as if both my lungs are involved." "Yes," Field said. "Well, I think I better go home and go to bed. I need to stop smoking and drinking for awhile." "Yes," the doctor said. "And I need medicine—some antibiotics and cough medicine." "I'll write the prescription," the doctor said. "While you're at it, please write something for pain. It hurts me every time I breathe. And I need to be re-examined to see how I'm doing." "I'll make an appointment in a

week." Ted went home to bed and ran his life by phone for a week. When he returned, his pneumonia had resolved. His parting remark was, "Well, Doctor, I guess when I first came in, I was trying to outfox you. If I didn't believe that what I did was the right thing for me to do, I'd think you outfoxed me."

In this story the doctor's focus was on the man and his illness, not just the disease. He was creative in his approach to enlisting Ted as a colleague in his own care. Ted created his own therapeutic plan, acceptable to him, and tailored to his particular needs. They cooperated and did not collude. They supported one another's growth. They gave love to one another.

THE COLLABORATIVE PARTNERSHIP

Increasing numbers of people want to be involved in their own health and medical care, to participate in the choices and decisions, and to be creative. They want their intelligence, common sense, and personal identity to be respected and acknowledged as valuable contributions to that process. Even if a person does not want all of those things, the prevalent person-doctor relationship is usually unsatisfactory. Much more desirable and effective is one in which person (patient) and doctor communicate effectively, are clear about expectations, and share responsibility and control. We are talking about partnerships as opposed to authoritarian or adversarial relationships.

In Table 15-1, four kinds of relationships are outlined. Two are partnerships; two are not. In the partnerships, physician and person share the responsibility and control for decision making. As the more informed expert, the physician's opinion often carries more weight. However, the person is always encouraged to gain further information and explore al-

TABLE 15–1   Control and Responsibility in Person-Doctor Relationships.

		Collaborative Partnership	Limited Partnership	Authoritarian	Adversarial
Responsibility	Doctor	when situation demands	more than patient	almost complete	none
	Patient	most of it most of the time	only some of time	very little	none
Control	Doctor	only if patient doesn't want it or is unable to take it	more than patient	almost complete	none
	Patient	most of it most of the time	only some of the time	very little	none

ternative modes of management. Some degree of shared responsibility/control ultimately defines partnership.

In a collaborative partnership, mutual trust and confidence build with time. The physician learns increasingly how you think, react, and make choices. She learns what your values are and your important opinions. Then if you are ever incapacitated by illness or accident, severe pain or fear, and are unable to participate, the doctor will make decisions that are in your best interest and closely reflect your own preferences. You can "surrender" control and responsibility with confidence and trust if dependence is necessary or desirable. The collaborative partnership sets the stage to minimize fear when an emergency occurs — shared control if you are not severely ill gives you confidence when you are.

This chapter has described some of the prevalent characteristics of PDR relationships in today's U.S. It has contrasted them with a glimpse of a much more caring, creative, and growing PDR where the concepts of love and partnership are predominant. In the next chapter, the PDR will be "dissected" to provide deeper understanding of the origins of present characteristics and how changes might be engineered to move toward the collaborative partnership ideal.

RESOURCES CHAPTER 15

Cassell, *The Healer's Art* (Cited in Chapter 6).
Preston, T. *The Clay Pedestal*. Seattle, WA: Madrona Press, 1981.

16

The Person-Doctor Relationship and How It Works (or Doesn't)

THE Person-Doctor Relationship (PDR) has four related and interdependent dimensions: control and responsibility, communication, expectations, and love and creativity. The quality of what goes on in each of these dimensions and how they interact determines both the kind of relationship that exists (adversarial, authoritarian, partnership) and its effectiveness. Since a partnership relationship with one's physician (or other health provider) is part of Personal Health Competence, this chapter seeks a deeper understanding of the four dimensions and how they function.

Quite apart from their commonality in business, partnerships occur in many other aspects of life. As a homespun example, here is a description of my mother and her grocer in the days before supermarkets.

My mother was a person who cared about food. She was a good cook. When my family moved to a new neighborhood, the first thing my mother did was get to know the tradesmen. The grocer she selected did not (and was not expected to) know all of her likes, dislikes, and idiosyncracies about meat and vegetables on her first or second visit to the store. She did, however, expect him to engage in a familiarization process over time. She expected him to talk with her about her food needs, and he expected to do that. Before long, the grocer did, in fact, know most of my mother's important tastes and preferences about the various foods she might order. Dorothea (as I called her) learned quickly about the grocer's strengths and weaknesses from her point of view. She improved her service by explaining what was satisfactory or unsatisfactory. The grocer said what he could and couldn't do. He also suggested good buys and alternatives when appropriate. She often asked his advice about what looked good that day. He often asked for feedback on how "the roast had been." They had a relationship, the success of which depended on good communication, clear expectations (including compatible goals), collaborative responsibility, and mutual support. It was occasionally creative, too. When "compromise" became necessary (as it often did when inflation or a bad growing season occurred), they both clearly understood it as a compromise. Occasionally they had "fights" or overt difficulties, but that was accepted as part of being clear with one another.

CONTROL AND RESPONSIBILITY

Control and responsibility determine who runs the show. The physician can assume an authoritarian, paternalistic role, giving the patient few, if any, real choices and responsibilities. This is a parent-child relationship. At the other side of the spectrum is the *collaborative partnership*, an adult-adult relationship. The patient is self-determining and involved.

With respect to control and responsibility, a number of factors ordinarily operate to the person's disadvantage. Most of us are conditioned to believe that the status and authority of physicans are pre-eminent. To the doctor's office we bring a set of reactions toward people with status and authority, which usually include feeling intimidated and inferior to a significant degree. On the basis of previous experience, some of us may not trust doctors or are scared. Further, when we go to a physician it is because something is troubling us; we are asking

the doctor to take care of us. This creates or increases a sense of dependence.

Also, the nature of the encounter itself is difficult. To obtain effective assistance you must often talk about personal matters and emotions. Secrets may be disclosed. The mind must undress, and most of the time your body as well. In the presence of some "busy" doctors, both must be done at once!

Add to these things the propensity of physicians (by training and professional culture) to be authoritarian, paternalistic, and sometimes condescending, and the stage is set for the commonest pattern of person-physician relatedness. It is accurately described as a parent-child relationship. In more elegant terms, it is an unequal relationship with the patient disadvantaged. The physician is in control — the physician has the authority and makes the decisions. Verbally and nonverbally, doctors repeatedly tell people "You will do what I say. You will come at my convenience. You will wait as long as I need you to." In short, patients are expected to be patient and submissive. Consequently they often abdicate responsibility and vest control of their care with the physician.

This outcome can be precipitated by either party: by an authoritarian physician or by a meek and submissive patient. In the vast majority of instances, however, both are operating — there is collusion. This is an important point. *While circumstances, attitudes, and past experiences frequently mitigate against the patient, creation of a parent-child situation still requires the person's participation.*

In each self-care class, there are always timid souls who complain about something their physician has done. We talk about ways in which a person might improve the situation by being more assertive. Despite repeated encouragement from peers as well as instructors, the help of a practice session in role playing, clear evidence that the unfortunate situation is continuing or has worsened, the party concerned does nothing new and continues to complain. This is collusion. The timid soul who is not colluding will either try to change things or stop complaining, thus signifying willingness to accept part of the responsibility for what is going on. Thus, even though some people *expect* (or will say they expect) something other than an authoritarian relationship, they collude with their physician to make that impossible.

These statements clearly reflect how importantly people regard clear and honest communication with their physician. Everyone who lists their priority expectations includes at least one that is directly related to communication. They are the same as or similar to the ones above.

A helpful and simple model of communication appears just below. Messages move in both directions through the channel. The direction of the message determines the receiver and the sender. In most patient-doctor encounters, the doc-

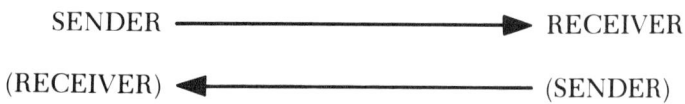

SENDER ——————————————▶ RECEIVER

(RECEIVER) ◀—————————————— (SENDER)

COMMUNICATION

Communication is vital. In a healthy relationship, communication grows in clarity and sophistication over time. People come to know each other's language, the process grows and matures, and the relationship blossoms. Poor communication hinders this.

The quality of communication is probably the main determinant of how well a single encounter or the ongoing process works. Good communication provides clarity and mutual respect. It *enables* other good things to happen. This is too often forgotten or, for the sake of short-term comfort, ignored.

I ask new students, "What are some of the important things you want of your physician?" Here are some replies:

"If he does not know what the problem is, he should say so."

"To be willing to understand the things (her patients are afraid or scared of). Speak with the patient as a friend and not anything less."

". . . be honest, as opposed to being evasive and protective with his patients . . ."

tor is perceived as the main sender and the patient as the receiver. This is true even during the interview, although the patient may do more of the talking. If things go well, however, the person and their physician intermittently reverse the direction of flow, occasionally even moving it in both directions at once.

Specific facts, information about feelings, and emotions may all be conveyed and understood. The nature, quality, and feelings of the flow are probably of equal or greater importance to the quality of the relationship than the time spent in communicating or the amount of information exchanged.

In this model, failures in communication may result from problems with you, problems with the physician, or problems (commonly referred to as "noise") within the channel. If the message is *clear* and the receiver can *hear*, there should be good transmission unless there is *noise* in the circuit.

In the typical patient-doctor relationship, communication is usually of poor quality. Frequently, for example, it flows mostly from doctor to patient. Something quite different is required — that is, a two-way exchange in which direction, spirit, and intensity may be modulated from moment to moment. Such "one-wayness" is the commonest communication problem in the person-doctor relationship, but other failures occur. A doctor's "busyness," attitudes, use of complicated words, and even "bedside manner," can all interfere seriously with good communication. A patient's attitudes ("Well, the doctor just keeps talking, but that's the way it is supposed to be.") or pain, worry, and anxiety can do the same.

"Busyness"

The physician seems very busy. The patient feels uncomfortable about taking more of the physician's time, and as a result does not say or ask something important.

Physician attitudes

The physician's attitudes, expressed verbally, nonverbally, or by implication, may belittle, intimidate, or anger the patient. These attitudes may also be conveyed by the doctor's tone of voice if it is pompous, condescending, or superior. No matter what the intent of the words, if they are delivered in these tones they are either not heard or cause unintended reactions. The following story is an excellent illustration of a physician, who had attitudes different from the patient's, trying to influence her decision — and of someone who would not be influenced.

Margaret is 35. Two years ago she had her first child, Peter, and she and her husband, Dieter, recently decided to have another. Margaret goes to a local Health Maintenance Organization (HMO) where she can state her preference for physicians. The pregnancy was established with certainty at four to five weeks. A nurse practitioner gave her the results of the lab tests, and explained that it was policy to do an amniocentesis on all mothers over 35[1]. Margaret replied that she and Dieter had discussed this possibility and had decided against it. When pressed for her reasons she said that even if Down's syndrome (Mongolism), was diagnosed, they would not have an abortion. The nurse practitioner's reaction was one of general displeasure. She argued with Margaret briefly, then gave her a booklet on birth defects.

Margaret saw a physician on her next visit. Looking at the chart he said, "I see you don't want to have an amniocentesis." Margaret explained as she had before. He then told her the statistics and argued that she and her husband were taking an unnecessary risk. Once again, Margaret repeated that she wasn't interested. Dr. Gaylord then said, "Well, it's your decision . . . but I do have a case right now of a woman who also refused and now, a month before delivery, it's clear that we have a fetus with multiple gross abnormalities." (Using isolated case experience in an attempt to persuade or intimidate someone to do what you suggest is common among physicians.) Margaret held her ground. She has chosen not to see that particular physician again.

Complicated words

The physician may use sophisticated or scientific language-words or concepts that you do not understand, sometimes called *jargon*: "ileitis" instead of inflammation of the small bowel, "immune response" instead of "your body's defenses."

Patient's attitudes

Patient attitudes may block or hinder effective communication. For example, a white man visiting a new doctor finds the doctor to be a woman or a black person (or even both!). This may generate conscious or unconscious reactions that lead to problems in communication.

1. Amniocentesis: amniotic fluid is drawn by needle from the placental sac. Analysis of the baby's skin cells (which have washed off) can then be done. There is low but definite risk of miscarriage following the procedure.

Worry or Pain

A patient may be too preoccupied with pain, or worry and frustration about being ill to hear or speak effectively. The physician may impart entirely correct and reliable information, but it is not "heard."

Finally, a most important reason for failure of communication is a clash in expectations. Commonly this is unrecognized. The next section covers the importance of this in greater detail.

EXPECTATIONS

"To put a greater emphasis on keeping well in the first place, rather than in treating problems *after* they arise."

". . . to be interested enough in me and my lifestyle to treat me as an individual."

"To give a complete explanation of medication use."

"To study diseases and alternate means of treating them — not necessarily involving medication; to be flexible in terms of the approach to treatment."

"To allow patients to collaborate in their own care; to share control."

These are not the words of a committee on how physicians should behave, but the responses of five different individuals in one self-care class to the question, "What is the most important expectation you have of physicians in practice?" They are not presented to fuel debate on what might be the most important answer. *Each is the most important answer to the individual who made it.* The responses illustrate the wide diversity in people's foremost expectations.

Expectations are the rules of the game: What do you think the rules are? What does the doctor think they are? Expectations define the behaviors that a person and doctor expect of one another. For effective transactions, high-priority ex-

pectations must be clear between parties and mutually attainable. Any great disparity in expectations must be reconciled. In the beginning of a relationship, unless they are discussed beforehand, the participants seldom see them as the same. People usually have greater and more varied expectations than the doctor has, but the doctor's expectations (like, "be on time," "listen to my recommendations and carry them out") usually become the operating rules, not the patient's. Part of becoming an effective consumer is learning how to change the game so that it is played by some of your rules, not always the physician's. Best of all, play by rules you both agree on!

Expectations are influenced by the *frame of reference* of each party. This includes both the person's and the physician's goals, their notion about what their work is together, their respective belief systems and values, and their styles of interaction. For example, a doctor (and patient) might see their work as primarily an "I help you — you help me" kind of affair in which the usual outcome is the prescription of medications. In contrast, another doctor (and person) might see the PDR as an "I'll help you take care of yourself — I'll take care of myself with your help." In that case, healing and curing strategies including alternatives would be thoroughly discussed before a decision. In both these examples, the views of doctor and patient are compatible. If the first doctor cared for the second patient, there could be trouble.

Or, consider a person whose general view of the PDR is one of collaboration and partnership. If she or he happens to select a physician who demands obedience to his recommendations and has little patience with questions or tolerance for alternative therapies, the relationship will be difficult and may fail, even though the physician follows up meticulously on problems, gives the patient all lab results, and does not hesitate to refer to a specialist when she or he doesn't know what the problem is. The following tale illustrates such a situation.

At age 30 Cynthia was attending college while also working. She and Joe had been married three years. Over several weeks, she became extremely tired and had a lot of hip and low back pain. She sought help for these from an osteopath and with exercise and stretching noted improvement. Then a facial rash erupted; the fatigue increased. Her family physician suspected Lupus Eruthematosis (LE). LE is a serious disease of many organ systems—kidney, lungs, joints, sometimes the brain, including the skin. Many patients are sensitive to sunlight, which can cause the rash, and in some of them the disease in the joints and kidneys can be activated by too much sun exposure.

Cynthia's physician confirmed the diagnosis with appropriate tests and referred her to a specialist. On the first visit Cynthia (with Joe as her advocate) told Dr. Lewis (a woman) that she wanted to be involved in the decision-making process and that she wanted significant control over what was going on. The physician seemed to support the idea. There was not a lot of discussion about what this meant. Appropriate medications were started and during the initial period of adjustment (which included overcoming her denial), Cynthia began a program of intensive general conditioning including bicycling and swimming. She did this to improve her general well-being and to counteract the noticeable muscle weakness she was experiencing. Her general well-being rapidly improved, and she gained a real sense of control. She became considerably stronger, felt encouraged and hopeful, and was genuinely proud of her accomplishment. After six weeks she saw Dr. Lewis who immediately became upset on noticing Cynthia's suntan. Cynthia began to report on her conditioning program, whereupon Dr. Lewis impatiently scolded her for being in the sun so much. When Cynthia said, "I really thought that if I strengthened my muscles, the disease would improve," Lewis replied abruptly that the LE was "over here" (moving her hands to one side of her body) and the other (meaning this desire to take care of her body and strengthen her muscles) "over there" (hands moving sharply to the opposite side).

Thus in seconds this physician discounted Cynthia's wonderful work. Furthermore, what Dr. Lewis told Cynthia is incorrect. In any illness, physical fitness is important for itself; the mental well-being and other positive psychological effects it engenders are equally invaluable, and in Cynthia's case, it could certainly counteract muscle weakness. This person took a wholistic approach to her illness. She was imprudent in overexposing herself to the sun but the physician overreacted, and, indeed, it is not certain that she had clearly educated Cynthia on this point in the first place. So the patient's approach and the accomplishments were discounted in one brief moment. Not helpful!

Some expectations are very explicit. It is not uncommon to see signs in doctor's waiting rooms that ask for prompt payment or clearly state that Medicaid will not be accepted. Unfortunately, in most physician-patient relationships the vast majority of expectations on both sides are unspoken and not explicit. This is confusing. To the extent that expectations can be clearly identified and stated, any relationship will benefit. The importance of this in securing an effective person-doctor relationship cannot be overemphasized. You and your doctor must both heed this advice or to a significant degree you will be engaging in a charade, not an effective transaction—and at your expense.

In the next chapter, on partnering skills, the process of clarifying expectations will be discussed further. There you will find a checklist (Table 17-1) compiled by a group of lay people.

LOVE AND CREATIVITY

This is the most difficult dimension of the PDR to express in factual terms. By definition it has a strong spiritual component. If present it can make the difference between a powerful growing experience and a relationship that is completely stuck and going through the motions. It is clear that if both participants in the relationship work together effectively on responsibility and control, communication, and expectations, this love and creativity dimension is more likely to manifest itself. However, even in satisfactory PDR's, this one is often conspicuous by its absence. It is, unfortunately, rare enough that it can be thought of as frosting on the cake. It requires an openness on the part of the physician not often seen, and either openness or desperation on the part of the patient. When it is absent, the people involved are not utilizing important parts of themselves in the transaction. It is best illustrated through contrasting examples.

When I was an intern, one of my weekly responsibilities was to spend half a day in the clinic to see people not sick enough to be admitted to the hospital or who had been discharged and returned to check their progress. Already exhausted, I often regarded clinic duty as an unwanted chore. A typical patient visit began with routine amenities. Then I would ask, "Well, how's it going?" The answer might be brief. If it was not, I would often cut it off by asking specific questions designed to monitor progress of the disease (I didn't think about illness then). "How's your breathing? How many pillows are you sleeping with? Any ankle swelling?" — questions for a patient with heart disease. When finished with the specific questions (and often I would write in the chart while the patient responded), I did whatever physical exam was indicated. We would then talk about medications, usually while I wrote the prescriptions. Frequent "okay's" would punctuate my instructions, but I didn't wait for responses. Seldom would I ask if the patient had questions. I might remonstrate about their doing this or that more faithfully. The patient left until the next visit — one week, two weeks, a month. When the encounter was over, no one had changed — not me, not the patient. When a year of encounters was over, the same was true. No one had grown.

In contrast to this scenario, I recently had the privilege of observing a vivid encounter between my friend Barry, who directs an Alcohol Recovery Unit, and a patient. Barry and I were sitting in a small conference room discussing the outcomes of a meeting just finished. Suddenly a counselor and a nurse entered the room with one of the patients, a woman in her fifties. I recognized her as a person who had been recently admitted to the unit to try seriously for the first time to control a combined addiction to alcohol and a number of tranquilizing and mood stimulating drugs. She was very agitated, and the nurse reported that Mrs. G had been taking part in the daily exercise sessions when she became so agitated that she "couldn't stand it" and left. Now she was crying, wringing her hands with great strength, and saying she was frightened and feeling anger. She sat in a chair, whereupon Barry, already sitting, pulled close enough to her so that he could lean forward and put his head within two inches of hers. Their initial conversation was held with their heads at that distance, foreheads almost touching, faces inclined toward the floor. She talked about how her anger (an emotion she had never really felt until that week) was bursting forth and how terrifying it was because she didn't know what she might do. Over the next ten minutes, she alternately expressed her anxiety in words, vigorously pounded both hands on her knees, cried, said she couldn't stand it, and then cycled through again. Verbally and non-verbally Barry facilitated this discharge of anger and its accompanying anxiety. He assured her that it was okay to feel what she was feeling, that he knew it was very painful, that he couldn't guarantee her that she wouldn't have to experience it again. Constantly underlying his words was the theme that "You are okay; this is part of you that you need to meet and learn about," and he reinforced all of these messages by making it completely clear that he felt okay about being close to her, touching her, and comforting her. He was both stating and acting out her okayness. After a few minutes, while she was still talking with great fear, he gently pulled her head forward onto his shoulder. She began to cry and seized his arm for its protection and comfort. Her sobbing punctuated the verbal exchange which continued some minutes while he held her head on his shoulder, she gripping his arm. As she became calmer, they pulled far enough apart to talk face to face with eye contact, but continued to hold hands. When it was clear that she was almost ready to leave the room they hugged, he 6'1" she about five feet tall. They hugged for at least 30 seconds, and I watched her become calmer and stronger.

Barry was entirely present for Mrs. G. She was wholly there with her fear and anger and trembling. During those minutes they were totally with one another. And healing began to occur. Barry let himself be loving; he let himself create the response which seemed to me as I observed, most helpful to her (Dr. Field did the same for Ted in the previous chapter). She came to the room desperate but also with amazing trust (based on their previous interviews) and allowed herself

to be available in ways that she had never allowed before. She created responses to life she had never created before. Many of them could not have happened without Barry's love during those moments and without his creativity through which that love was expressed.

This story also illustrates the importance of appropriate physical contact between a person and their doctor. This is an aspect of interaction that is neglected by most physicians. It has become a casualty of high-technology medical practice. The reassurance value and aid to healing (not curing disease necessarily, but healing illness) of simply touching patients with the hands is again being recognized. Yet physicans do not employ appropriate touching. Hugging can be even more therapeutic if done at the appropriate time and if free of sexual overtones.

This powerful scenario was moving, dramatic, and highly effective in meeting Mrs. G's needs. While unfortunately rare in the practice of medicine, counseling, nursing, or practices of other health providers, an interaction of this kind is not unique or idiosyncratic. In the context of a partnership, this degree of presence, by both physician and patient, is possible far more often than it now occurs.

Good communication, shared responsibility and control, clarity of expectations, and love with creativity are the critical elements of strong person-doctor relationships. While it is not easy, with attentiveness and work, these elements can be crafted and used with the same power we have just witnessed.

Returning briefly to my mother's relationship with the grocer: it was certainly not as complicated psychologically as most person-doctor ones. However, it had the same important features. Control and responsibility were shared. It was meaningful to Dorothea that one person have her continuing business and that he feel important to her. In a similar way, the grocer wanted both my mother's business and her trust and friendship. They were true colleagues. It was an unstuck creative relationship. They helped one another grow and in that sense gave love — it was truly a collaborative partnership.

Attention to the same dimensions can enrich any person's relationship with their physician. In the next chapter the beliefs and skills that will help you develop and maintain a partnership with your physician are presented.

RESOURCES CHAPTER 16

Cassell. *The Healer's Art* (Cited in Chapter 6).

Sharf, B.F. *The Physician's Guide to Better Communication.* Dallas, Texas: Scott, Foresman and Company, 1984.

Sagov, S.E. with Brodsky, A. *The Active Patient's Guide to Better Medical Care.* New York: McKay, 1976.

17

The Beliefs and Skills of Health Partnership

BEING an effective partner with your physician or other health provider does not just happen. It requires believing that the idea makes sense, is feasible, and will provide significant advantage for you. Then it is necessary to acquire a set of skills that will enable and strengthen your partnership efforts. The beliefs and skills you need to be a successful health partner are presented in this chapter. They are another key aspect of Personal Health Competence.

THE PERSONAL BELIEFS THAT UNDERLIE HEALTH PARTNERING

To be an effective health partner, most people need to move from an authoritarian relationship with their physician to a more collaborative one. There are five personal beliefs critical to such a change. If they seem familiar, it is because they are derived from the alternative health beliefs that are presented earlier in this book.

1. I am responsible for my health and well-being, not my doctor.
2. I am capable of knowing more about myself than anyone else can know.
3. What I do with respect to my health and wellness is ultimately far more important than what my doctor does.
4. Physicians are not omnipotent; they do not always have the best answers.
5. I can become an effective working partner with my physician for both maintenance of my health and handling of medical problems as they arise.

172

A number of the stories presented in foregoing chapters illustrate the fundamental importance of the first belief. It is a basic premise of this book.

Belief number two likewise needs little amplification. Each of us has access to information, feelings, and ideas about ourselves that no one else can fathom until we recall or become aware of them. The self-appraisal in Chapter Two is intended to help you do this for the past and present. With every new illness or problem, you will be the most valuable and prolific source of data in relation to what is going on. You are the best source of emotional data about yourself, the only one who can put certain facts in correct juxtaposition, and (of great value but little used) your own notions about what is wrong with you and what is needed may frequently be better than the doctor's.

The third belief is illustrated by Figure 17-1.

your diet, not smoke, exercise, fasten your seat belt, and promote your own emotional stability and health.

"Physicians are not omnipotent"—belief 4. Indeed they are not. It humbles and excites me to remember all the times that people named their own problem—sometimes when I hadn't thought of it. Many also suggested remedies that might work better than one I prescribed. Until I became wiser, I often got defensive. Now I listen because so often they are right. Any honest physician can give numerous examples of times when "the patient knew best."

The last belief in the list logically follows from the rest and needs no further discussion. It's realization does depend on gaining the skills of health partnering.

Merely reading these five beliefs will not automatically incorporate them into your belief system, but having them in front of you and referring to them periodically as you practice the skills will be

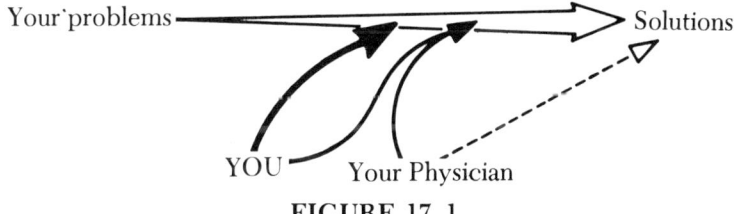

FIGURE 17-1.

In the diagram, the thickness of the lines is proportional to the actual input from the source it represents. *What you do yourself is most important*—not for every problem, but over the years. What you and your physician do together is next in importance. What the physician does without your participation has the least impact.

The validity of this attitude is powerfully illustrated by data already used in the assessment chapter. The important risk factors for the major killing, mutilating, and disabling problems are under your control. Your doctor may make suggestions, but it is you that has to change

extremely helpful. As you become more accomplished in the skills, the attitudes will seem more real. As you change the nature of the relationship with your physician, the attitudes will change, sometimes in advance of the skills, sometimes because you have mastered a certain skill. You may already have some of these attitudes without realizing it. Simply seeing them in writing may turn out to be an "aha" for you.

THE SKILLS OF HEALTH PARTNERSHIP

The skills that will be helpful in your "health partnering" endeavors are:

- clearly describing problems or illness — telling your story
- clarifying expectations
- using an advocate
- considering alternatives to drugs and surgery
- obtaining second opinions
- being assertive (about all of the above and in general)
- being critical: guarding against quackery
- the wise use of medications

Some physicians still balk when alternatives are suggested, and some will be at least mildly defensive when you request a second opinion. Nevertheless, your competence in these skills will generally enhance rapport, communication, and collaboration between you and your physician, above and beyond the direct benefits gained from the skills themselves.

Clearly describing problems or illness (telling your story)

This skill sharpens communication and saves time. To clearly describe what you experience, pay close attention to the following:

1. Location of the complaint. It is usually easy to locate pain or other physical discomfort. With emotions it is also often possible to identify a part of the body from which the sensation seems to come. If it moves or goes (radiates) to other parts of the body, this is also important.
2. When it began; when it last recurred.
3. How long it lasts, both initially and with subsequent appearances.
4. Is the problem steady or does it cycle from better to worse to better?
5. Is there any circumstance or stimulus (like a particular food for example) that seems to make it start, get worse, or improve?

6. What is its quality? Sharp, dull, pleasant, unpleasant?
7. How strong or intense is the complaint? Remember that not only pain has intensity; a cough does also, as does fear.
8. What other sensations or symptoms accompany the main complaint?
9. Have you had this before? If so, is it the same or different? How was it treated?
10. What changes or differences have you had in your life lately (including emotional or stressful ones) that might be associated with this symptom in some way?
11. Are you taking medications? If so, what?
12. Do you have any personal or work habits that might be related to the problem (like smoking)?
13. Has anything unusual been happening good or bad: stress/successes, strains/pains, joys/jilts?
14. Is there anything else that seems important?
15. What has been done for the problem: treatment, tests, with what results?

The skill of telling your story is improved by keeping a journal or practicing with a friend. In real situations it is desirable to use the above checklist.

To say, "I have a stomach ache" is one thing. But the following is much more helpful: "I have a very sharp pain about two inches above my belly button. It lasts a few seconds and happens once or twice an hour. It occured for the first time yesterday and has continued since, though it didn't seem to keep me awake or occur during the night. It happens only when I'm standing, and is better when I'm lying down. I have not had any nausea or vomiting or diarrhea with the pain." It is not hard to learn how to describe your own pain (or any other symptom) with similar exactitude.

Clarifying Expectations

As stated earlier, expectations are the rules of the game, what you think the rules are, and what the doctor thinks they are. Regardless of whether or not your physician is clear about his or her expectations, it is vital that you clarify yours. Stop now in your reading, and write down in your notebook three or four of the expectations that you have of your physician.

When you have made your list, take a look at Table 17-1, which was compiled by one class of self-care students. It is a *useful checklist* for negotiating an agreement with a physician because it reminds people of things they might otherwise forget and helps prioritize expectations. This is extremely important.

TABLE 17-1   One Group's Expectations of Their Doctor.
_____

 1. Listens
 2. Informs and explains
    A. What's wrong
    B. Why she does what she does
    C. About medications, including side effects
    D. Lab results
 3. Itemizes bills
 4. Direct and open
 5. Not superior, is respectful
 6. Allows patients to collaborate in their own care, to share control
 7. Responds to me as a person
 8. Acknowledges my feelings
 9. Honest, says "I don't know," refers to a specialist when necessary
10. Hopeful
11. Relaxed, takes time
12. Models what she preaches
13. Open to alternatives
14. Interested in health over long haul, not just taking care of illness
15. Provides continuity, follow up

To continue the process of defining your expectations, choose three or four that are most important and make the statements as clear as possible. Remember to include expectations about being treated as a person and about utilizing your other partnering skills (e.g., you expect the doctor to help you keep your self-health record and to look at it when you bring it to the office). Finally, make it an important expectation that you and the physician will periodically review expectations.

Using an Advocate

The principles involved in learning to use an advocate have been discussed in Chapter 11. In training your advocate, make sure she or he understands your expectations of the doctor. To check this ask your advocate to recite those expectations to you. It is essential that your advocate clearly understands your position, your philosophy, and your values.

Before visiting your physician, discuss with your advocate: why you are going (what your goals and questions are, what you want to come away with), your philosophy about procedures that might be suggested by the doctor, and previous problems you may have had interacting with the same physician. Whether your advocate should actually accompany you to the physician can be dealt with on a time-by-time basis. However, an advocate needs to see your physician in action once or twice a year. For difficult problems, it may be best that they go each time, but this depends on how you and the physician are progressing with the partnership. Don't forget, if you intend to use an advocate, one expectation to be clarified with your doctor is that you be allowed to have your advocate in the examining room with you.

Considering Alternatives to Drugs and Surgery

Chapter 20 will discuss the "knee-jerk" mentality that governs the overuse of drugs and surgery in therapy. It is sufficient here to point out that almost any condition probably has more than one acceptable mode of treatment. Some-times all of the acceptable modes involve medications or surgery, but many times they do not. So this skill first involves remembering to remember to ask about alternatives. The next step is to acquire the necessary information. Read, talk to informed people, or call or write to consumer advocate offices or consumer clearing houses (see Resources).

Here is a short list of common medical problems for which acceptable alternatives may be used (Table 17-2). I say "may" because it is essential to remember that an alternative may or may not work in a given individual or that it may in some instances be wiser to proceed with standard therapy.

- When advised to have a certain kind of treatment or surgery for which reasons, appropriateness, and safety are uncertain.
- *Anytime* major elective surgery or other life threatening intervention has been suggested.
- Inability to understand the physician.

Are second opinions a good idea? Definitely. Anytime there is uncertainty about a decision, mistrust of the physician, or poor understanding, get one. Their cost is usually well worthwhile.

How do you ask for one? If your doctor is quite authoritarian, it can be difficult. However, second opinions are common enough so that a request for one

TABLE 17-2.

Medical Problem	Accepted Standard Therapy	Alternative Therapy
Coronary artery disease	by-pass surgery	diet, regular exercise, weight loss, blood pressure control
Moderately elevated blood pressure (diastolic reading 100–105)	pills (usually at least 2 kinds)	salt reduction, exercise, weight control, relaxation, meditation
Adult onset diabetes	oral hypoglycemic agents (for some cases)	weight loss, exercise
Metastatic cancer	chemotherapy	natural food diet, communication skills (interactive skills) and guided imagery with or without chemotherapy
Upper respiratory infections	over the counter drugs, antibiotics	fluids, rest, no medications
Constipation	pills, mineral oil, other laxatives	high fiber diet, dried fruits, vegetarian diet

Obtaining Second Opinions

This skill involves recognizing those situations in medical work where another opinion about diagnosis or therapy may be important. They include:

- A serious or potentially serious problem for which the diagnosis is uncertain.

is unlikely to cause lasting difficulty. The important thing is to be clear. Say, "I want another opinion." *Do not ask whether the doctor thinks another opinion would be a good idea.* In choosing the person to whom you will go for a second opinion, *it is not a good idea to go to someone your doctor suggests.* It is hard for doctors to disagree with friendly colleagues who also refer patients to them. If you don't know who to see and if your friends (particularly physicians, paramedics, nurses, or pharmacists) cannot advise you, call the medical society (an excellent step to take in any case), and explain that you want a second opinion. They can probably furnish the names of a number of people to contact. Your health insurance company should be willing to do the same.

What should you do if the second opinion is different from the first? Either get a third opinion or return to your family physician (presuming she is not the one who gave the original opinion). In either case, take all of the records and written opinions with you and discuss them directly with the doctor. You must weigh your own feelings very highly. If the opinions are divided, it is important that you choose the path that feels the most comfortable and safest to you.

On Being Assertive

Even if you have planned well and are clear about your needs and expectations, you will still need to be assertive to attain them. It is important that your preparation make you *specifically purposeful.* Enter the arena with clarity about what you want, not just the vague sense that you want something. This greatly increases the odds of a successful and satisfying encounter, as opposed to one that is frustrating or angering. Here are some suggestions that can help you be effectively assertive:

1. *Role play the visit in advance.* Have a friend or family member (one who knows the doctor) play the part of the doctor. Say what your expectations are, overcome interruptions, make the doctor stay longer to answer those unanswered questions.
2. *Rehearse the essential lines aloud.* This may be part of the role playing,

or done alone, if necessary. "Doctor, your language is too complicated for me; please explain that again." "I want to know the name of this medication and its side reaction." "Is there another way this condition could be treated than with medication?" *You must rehearse aloud.* Hear yourself and practice the lines, each time becoming more and more assertive.
3. *Know your top priorities,* then have fantasies about achieving them. Picture getting what you expect from the doctor, being assertive and clear as you do it. Spend time on this—it is helpful. Do not dwell on fantasies in which you are patronized, scolded, put down, and in which you do not attain your expectations.
4. *Be clear, clean, and concise.* Clarity: know what you want to say and say it as clearly as possible. Clean: do not mix your main message with other concerns. For example, if you are unhappy with your physician about the last bill, but are in the office today to discuss changing a medication, don't say, "Well, Dr. Evinrude, I want to change my blood pressure medication, if we can talk about it for less than a hundred bucks." Concise: say everything as briefly as possible. Time is always of concern to your physician.
5. *Reserve anger and indignation as last resorts.* Effective assertiveness is not the same as being angry. Occasionally, the expression of dissatisfaction and anger may be necessary to achieve your purposes. Most often, however, firmness, a strong tone of voice, and a confident air will be sufficient.

Being Critical: Guarding Against Quackery

Health and wellness is a welcome and blossoming industry today in the United

States. Hospitals, health spas, small business, and publishing houses are producing reading materials, listening and looking materials, and programs.

Also, in any health or women's magazine, most newspapers and even in conservative newsmagazines, one finds reports of new treatments that are not pharmaceuticals or surgery. Some are patently sensational, and others evenly presented and apparently supported by good evidence.

These programs, products, and treatments vary widely in quality and effectiveness. It often may be difficult to tell which may be safe and effective and which may only be exploiting an increasingly popular market.

Here are some principles to help distinguish legitimate health care from chicanery.

- Anytime someone advertises or states that their product is the cure for *everything* from warts to intermenstrual bleeding, avoid it
- Watch out for products that "always work"; such claims are unlikely and suggest deliberate attempts to deceive; only a few products work all of the time
- If the remedy is taken internally, be sure it is not harmful; ask your doctor, ask your pharmacist; call the regional poison center (regional ones are better than local ones); go to the library and read about it
- If the product has been around awhile it is less likely to be fraudulent
- Talk to people who have had the treatment; ask for names of those who didn't fare as well
- The smooth talker who doesn't give direct answers and makes great claims is the one to watch; if people are not evasive and admit that their thing sometimes doesn't work, they are much more likely to be okay

- If advertising is found in reputable places, the product is more likely to be reliable
- When using a treatment about which you have some doubts, monitor your body carefully for new symptoms, changes in the ways your body functions, rashes, itching and other abnormal signs.

Using Medicines Safely and Effectively

While the wise use of medications is definitely a health partnering skill, it is vitally important for *all* people whether or not they want a partnership with their doctors. We are a substance-oriented society. We depend on tobacco, alcohol, and medications (all multibillion dollar industries) to provide us with relief, distraction and rest from our difficulties and problems, or with entertainment to relieve our boredom. We think every problem has a solution in the form of a pill, injection, or other "magic" remedy. Advertisers would have us believe that any "symptom" calls for an external agent. Most patients feel gypped if they leave the physician's office without a prescription.

As we gain the potentially beneficial effects of these materials, we often forget they are short-lived and that many medications are habit forming. Like illegal street drugs, these lawful substances all have potential for being unhealthy and lethal. Even those that are not addicting are still potentially dangerous, some very dangerous. *There is no such thing as an entirely safe medicine.*

After you have tried to answer the following questions (guesses are fine), study the answers. They may astound you.

1. How many dollars are spent each year in the United States on prescription drugs?
2. How many dollars are spent on nonprescription medications?

3. What kinds of medicines are most commonly prescribed?
4. What percentage of patients seen in the office does the average physician write at least one prescription for?
5. What percentage of all hospitalized patients have an "unwanted consequence of drug administration" (doses omitted, wrong medication, severe side effects, allergic or hypersensitivity reactions, antagonism of another drug)?

Over $15 billion are spent each year on prescription drugs and another $3–4 billion for cheaper nonprescription, over-the-counter medications.

Of the 20 medications most commonly prescribed in office practice, six are antibiotics (totaling 41,000,000 new prescriptions), six are used for heart disease or high blood pressure, three are for pain, inflammation, or both (as in arthritis), two are for immunizations, and one is insulin for diabetes. The two remaining ones are valium, at 6,000,000 new prescriptions a year, and tagamet, at 5,400,000 new prescriptions per year.[1] Antibiotics are used to treat infections but are not effective against viral illnesses like flu, most sore throats and the common cold. Blood pressure medications are often used before trying alternative therapies (and in severe high blood pressure they should be). Tagamet is effective in the treatment of ulcer disease, a condition caused in most cases by anxiety and tension. Valium is a "minor" tranquilizer with addictive potential. It is prescribed for anxiety, tension, and stress.

Seventy-five percent of all patients leaving doctors' offices have been given at least one prescription. Twenty percent of all hospitalized patients have an "unwanted consequence of drug administration."

1. National Ambulatory Medical Care Survey, 1981, U.S. Department of Health and Human Services, Public Health Service.

Most leading prescription medications are prescribed far in excess of their usefulness. Antibiotics are one example, but there are many others (6000 different medicines are available by prescription). In the U.S. there are 30,000 nonprescription medicinal products. Many, of course, are merely the same substances or mixtures under different names. Some of these also can be habituating or addicting. Most have potentially troublesome or dangerous allergic potential or side effects and must be used with care. As one example, cold medications are greatly overused.

Furthermore, it is now obvious that aerobic exercise, relaxation, other stress management techniques, and good nutrition can prevent most headaches, control or eliminate anxiety and sleeplessness, relieve tension, and control the effects of many psychosomatic illnesses. These are the problems for which valium, librium, and other potentially addicting psychotropic drugs are prescribed. Physicians are wrong not to consider alternatives with their patients. Patients are not being responsible when they demand such medications without exploring alternatives first. The leading drug addiction in this country today is probably not to heroin, cocaine, or other "street drugs," but to tranquilizers like valium and librium. It is an addiction rooted almost invariably in the physician's prescription pad, with the complicity of the patient.

The following story is typical.

SARAH

Sarah Grange was married at 23, a year after finishing college, to Tom, who soon became a successful small business executive. In the first ten years of marriage the couple had four children, entertained frequently as part of Tom's work, and had an active social life outside the home. At 37 Sarah developed mild arthritis, which required aspirine for control.

Her alcohol consumption was steady but never excessive on a social basis. When her arthritis progressed, she was advised to take a stronger anti-inflammatory agent that she used along with the aspirin. As her children grew older and progressed to college, Sarah found herself with more time to herself, bored, and having frequent headaches. Her doctor discussed these superficially and prescribed valium. At first she took this medication in small doses and felt some relief from her anxiety and boredom as well as her headache. After a couple of months she increased the dose on her own and took them on a daily basis. After a year (she never had trouble getting the drug renewed by calling her physician's office) she was taking about 80 mg a day and was feeling quite listless in the morning. A friend suggested she try some dexedrine ("speed") to counteract that feeling in the morning and became her supplier for that drug. It was a matter of time before she was taking that on a regular basis also. Sarah continued in this pattern for three more years, still taking aspirin and butazolidine for arthritis, dexedrine, and valium, the latter 80–100 mg/day. It was not until she developed some breast nodules for which she was hospitalized that anything changed. Fortunately, she was seen in consultation by a new physician who seriously questioned what was happening. Afraid herself by this time, she was honest about the extent of her habit and with Dr. Newcomb's help and encouragement entered a drug recovery and rehabilitation program. Within a month she was drug free (including the butazolidine) and participating in group therapy. A year later she was cheerful, outgoing, excercising regularly, back in school working for an advanced degree and completely free of all medications.

GUIDELINES FOR THE SAFE USE OF MEDICATIONS

Despite the facts cited above, medicines are essential and important in the management of many illnesses. The following guidelines can increase their margin of safety. Read them and ask what you

and your family do and don't do. After the guidelines is a medication list. List all the medications in the house that you decide *not* to throw out, and fill in the rest of the information as completely as possible.

1. Know all your medications, both prescription and over-the-counter. For each medicine you use, learn from your physician, your pharmacist, or a good reference book (see Resources) all of the following: (a) what it is supposed to do; (b) the recommended dosage, time schedule, and best time (if any) to take it (e.g., before meals); (c) how long it takes to work; (d) restrictions or limitations — anything you should or shouldn't do while taking it; (e) risks and side effects; (f) price; (g) whether it should be taken until used up (antibiotics unless side reactions occur) or stopped when you feel better (pain medication).

2. Keep a list (see Figure 17-2) of your medications, their dosage, and how often to take them. Also include purpose of the medicine, side effects, and possible cross reactions with other medications. The names and expiration date should also be on the label of each container. If they are not, ask the pharmacist to put them there.

3. *Always* read the label of any medication, prescribed or nonprescribed. If there is anything you do not understand, ASK.

4. If you skipped a dose (or think you have), do not try to catch up. Continue on your usual schedule. As a rule, it is much riskier to take extra medications than to miss one or two doses.

5. Keep all medications out of the reach and sight of children.

6. Make sure that any physician, den-

tist, or other person who prescribes medicine for you knows what other medications you are taking and whatever allergic reactions you have to medicines, i.e., nausea, hives, anaphylaxis.

7. If definitely allergic to a medication, do not take it again except under careful observation or supervision, and not even then unless the indications for it are very strong.

8. If you believe any medicine may be causing a side effect or allergic reaction, stop taking it and talk to your pharmacist or physician as soon as possible.

9. Never increase the dose of a prescription unless you have discussed this ahead of time with your physician or pharmacist.

10. Don't use medicines that were prescribed for other people. You never know what's in those bottles.

11. With essential medicines that must be taken indefinitely (such as insulin, blood pressure medications, or certain heart drugs like Digoxin) make sure to refill prescriptions ahead of time so you are not caught empty-bottled. If no refills have been authorized, call your doctor's office.

12. Keep medications only in the original container.

13. Operate on the premise that drug advertising doesn't tell the whole story. Never accept new claims for a drug without identifying the facts from one or two other sources. Make sure your sources are reputable. Read your books, read the inserts and labels, ask your pharmacist.

Surveying Your Medications and Starting a Medications List

Survey and clean out your medicine cabinets, refrigerators, bureaus, and any other nooks and crannies where medicines are kept. Look in all the logical places and line up those medicines. How many are there? What is their average use? Given the guidelines on previous pages, what are your reasons for keeping them around? Do you know what they are all for?

Among those that you have collected, there will be some that you can throw away without further consideration. Such drugs include those that are old enough to be unreliable, not well labeled, or haven't been used in a long time. Get rid of them; put them down the toilet to avoid the possibility that your children or someone else's will find and consume them. There will probably be some which you or other members of the household are using at the present time. Keep those, of course, and enter them properly on your medication list. This leaves a bunch you are not sure about. You're not using them now, but they're "fairly new," "still mostly full," and you're pretty sure that, if you keep them around long enough, "they'll get used" and save you a lot of money in the process. If you are sure what something is and are likely to need it again (like pain or allergy medications), it is okay to keep them until the expiration date. If they are antibiotics do not keep them around unused. Enter any of those you keep on the list, even if you only have a few medications in the home, list them.

The form shown in Figure 17-2 is one way your list might be designed. It is self-explanatory. You may not be able to fill out all the columns for each medication, but for any that you are taking at the present time, it is important to get any missing information as soon as possible and fill it in.

At the Risk of Repetition

A few final words about medications. Before taking a new medicine prescribed by

FIGURE 17-2   Medication List.

Name of Medication	Date Purchased	What it is for	Prescribed Dose	Potential Toxicity	Effects on Me

your physician, make sure you know *what it is supposed to do, what its side effects might be,* and how likely they are to occur (antihistamines make practically *everyone* drowsy). Equally important, ask your doctor *if there is an alternative way* of managing the condition that might be tried before you take the medication(s). Then, and only then, make a decision about what to do. If in your relationship with your physician, you don't change anything else, *do* demand that he properly inform you about recommended medications and any potential alternatives. It is a matter of sickness and health.

Similarly, when you are tempted to buy an over-the-counter drug (often a drug mixture), ask yourself the same questions. Is there another alternative (such as humidifying your room for chronic nasal congestion instead of taking Sine-Aid?) If not, what do you believe this over-the-counter medicine will do, why do you want to try it, what side effects does it have?

The right medication, wisely chosen, for the right purpose may be an important treatment for you to use. But don't let our medication-oriented medical care system use you. Be the boss. Control your own therapy.

This chapter has stated five personal

health beliefs and described a number of skills that are the basis for effective health partnering. The beliefs support the primacy and potential competence of any individual in the care of his or her health. When learned, the skills provide the tools for being personally competent in health partnering, the process of working effectively with one's physician (or other provider) to maintain personal health and heal illness. The skills can obviously be practiced in a number of different situations and the next series of chapters will describe some of those.

RESOURCES CHAPTER 17

Ardell. *High Level Wellness* (See General Resources).

Graedon, J. and Graedon, T. *The People's Pharmacy* (Books 1 & 2). New York: Avon, 1976 and 1980. Graedon's books are well informed, lively, and speak to the main problems that people need to be aware of and educated about with respect to drugs. I always start with these books when interested in learning more about a drug.

Holvey. *Merck Manual.* (See General Resouces).

Kiester. *Better Homes and Gardens New Family Medical Guide* (See General Resources).

Physician's Desk Reference. Oradell, NJ: J.E. Angel, publisher, Medical Economics,

Co., 1984. The standard office manual for drug information. Almost too detailed, but since companies are required to mention all known side effects and interactions it is one of the definitive resources.

Ryan and Travis. *Wellness Workbook* (See General Resources).

Sagov. *The Active Patient's Guide to Better Medical Care* (Cited in Chapter 16).

Sehnert. *How to be Your Own Doctor (Sometimes)* (See General Resources).

Silverman, H.M. and Simon, G.I. *The Pill Book. The Illustrated Guide to the Most Prescribed Drugs in the United States.* New York: Bantam Books, 1979. Information on hundreds of the commonest prescription drugs including side effects, with illustrations of about 500 of them so that you can identify unknown pills. Also has a useful table of drug interactions.

18

Finding and Getting Started with a New Physician (Or Starting Over with Your Old One)

A COMMON question in these days of high geographic mobility (20 percent of U.S. families move each year) and changing consumer expectations is, "How do I find a new doctor?" This chapter will help you apply knowledge and skills gained in previous chapters to both the task of finding likely candidates and deciding whether or not they are the person you want. The second set of strategies may also be used to infuse new energy into an existing but tired person-doctor relationship.

SOME CRITERIA USED FOR CHOOSING PHYSICIANS ARE LESS HELPFUL THAN COMMONLY THOUGHT

There are a number of criteria often advocated for choosing physicians that I consider of minimal value. For predicting the performance of large numbers of physicians, they are of some use. However, in terms of assessing the performance and competence of a single doctor, they are virtually meaningless.

First, a physician's medical school says nothing about competence. Although a place like Harvard may produce more good physicians than the University of Kansas (I don't really know) his or her school tells you nothing about a particular individual. All schools produce competent, less competent, and incompetent people, and quality depends more on the individual than the school they attend. This statement is probably less true in the case of graduates of foreign medical schools, but it still applies.

Second, whereas the length and quality of training after medical school is important, the number of years alone can be deceiving. For some people and their particular set of problems, a family physician or specialist in internal medicine with only two years of extra training may be a more compatible and effective physician than one with five.

Third, certification by a specialty board (like the American Board of Internal Medicine) is often overvalued. Most specialty board examinations are much more a test of ability to prepare for an examination than of competence as a physician. They do help safeguard against outright fakes, but plenty of poor doctors have board certification. Membership in the county medical society or on a hospital staff is, in some communities, probably the best (though by no means sure) safeguard against the charlatan. You must have a degree, a license, and references to join.

Fourth, membership in "learned" societies is overrated. Most professional societies operate somewhat like fraternities. In any case, the criteria for membership usually has little to do with *competence as a practitioner* of medicine. The same goes for VIPs in academic or non-academic medicine. Although it is true that medical VIPs are "dedicated," they are also *very* busy. Often their main concerns are with research, medical administration, or medical politics. The time that they have for patients and for their own continuing education suffers thereby.

Finally, let's consider that honored quality, "bedside" (or "deskside") manner. Many physicians have cultivated a pleasant and cheerful manner with patients. A significant number of these use their "manner" as a way of separating or distancing themselves from patients, their suffering and their concerns. A veneer of joviality is often substituted for genuine concern. A dismissal of significance, "don't you worry about that,

okay?" too often blocks communication. So be alert. Sincerity, honesty with your own feelings, and attentive listening are the gold currency of interaction — beware of false substitutes!

COMPILING A LIST OF PROSPECTS

Before even beginning to compile a list, it is essential to clarify and prioritize your expectations. Use the checklist in Chapter 17. Decide which expectations you won't compromise at all and which you will compromise to some extent. This will be useful when you are talking to other people about the kind of physician you are looking for. When you are ready, a number of strategies are useful to develop a list of names. Usually you have to use several strategies to get even a short list of available physicians.

1. Find out from your local library or pharmacist whether the County Medical Society or other community organization has published a doctor's directory. Even if available, they vary in quality and degree of usefulness. From a good one, you can get a lot of help in terms of types of practice, office hours, partnership status, on-call arrangements, and hospital affiliations of the doctors in the community.

2. In most places the County Medical Society keeps a list of physicians who accept new patients. This provides you with a set of physicians who are ostensibly available. For those, the society's secretary or executive officer should be able to tell you age, sex, length of time in practice, and type of practice, but will offer little, if any, assistance insofar as quality goes. It is very unlikely they will recommend one practitioner over others of the same specialty, though there's no harm in asking.

3. More names may be obtained from friends, the local pharmacist, and any nurses or physicians that you may know socially or to whom you were referred by your previous physician for advice. In talking to these people, remember not to just ask, "Do you know a good doctor?" or "Tell me who I should go to," but *speak specifically from your list of high priority expectations.* In this way, your friends and other contacts will have a description of the physicians you are looking for. Then they can be a lot more helpful. Most Americans understand that an athlete does not get drafted by the major leagues because a couple of scouts think,"He's really good." They are drafted on the basis of specific abilities (speed, strength, agility) that are carefully scored in the scouting process. Your expectations allow you to be similarly specific when choosing a physician.

From these four strategies, you will have a list of names. Although you may have only one possibility you will probably have two or three. If the list is longer than three pare it down.

THE INITIAL INTERVIEW

Now it is time to arrange interviews with one or more of the people on your list. This may not be easy because doctors are not used to people coming just to "check them out." It is essential to make this appointment at a time *when you are well.* If you try and do other things such as having the doctor check your nose which has been bothering you, either you or the physician can make that the main order of business. So, when you call, tell the nurse or receptionist that you need 15–20 minutes of the doctor's uninterrupted time. Say that you are willing to come at a time other than usual office hours if necessary, like just before or after regu-

lar office hours. Make it clear that you expect to pay for this special appointment. To help you prepare for the interview consider rehearsing the scene at home with a friend or family member playing the role of the doctor. If it is with someone who actually knows the physician, all the better. They can imitate mannerisms and ways of speaking.

As you are waiting to see the doctor, remember that a first meeting requires certain amenities and more cautious pacing than you might employ at a later time. When you are face to face with the physician, open the conversation firmly. Do not be negative or apologetic. Don't say, "I'm sorry to take up your time like this." Use a positive, assertive introduction:

"Dr. Klein, I'm George Parks. I'm new in town and in the process of trying to find a physican for the family. I know that it's probably unusual for someone to come and interview you, to sort of see how they like you and the sound of your practice but basically that's why I'm here, and I really appreciate your willingness to do this with me." Then give Dr. Klein a chance to respond before continuing. When he's ready, swing right into the expectations: "Dr. Klein, I've thought a lot about the traits I would like to have in a physician and his practice, and I'd like to begin by telling you what the highest priority items are." And you're off.

If this interview is for the purpose of revitalizing a tired relationship, the conversation might begin with, "Dr. Smith, I'm here today to talk about our relationship," or, "Doc, I feel that it's time we clarified our expectations of one another."

The physician's initial response may be calm and interested or jocular, angry, or evasive. He may become uncomfortable. Don't be put off. All of these responses give you data to work with.

Be as clear and concise as possible. Express your expectations positively. Use words like *want* and *expect*. Do not get caught in the trap of asking the physician whether he *can* or *can't* do certain things. It is not harmful or distracting to have things written down ahead of time or at least to have notes for yourself. As an example, here's what one person wrote.

My health is a two-person problem — mine and my doctor's. I'm an expert on me, he's an expert on my body functions. If I can communicate what's bothering me, I expect him to analyze and explain what could be the causes of the problem. Then, I'd like both of us to agree on a program to alleviate or correct the source of the problem. I dislike treating symptoms. I do not burden my doctor with every ache or pain so that when I do seek his help, I expect prompt attention . . . I like doctors to be interested enough in me and my life-style to treat me as an individual. I also like doctors who emphasize good health habits as a preventative to medical problems.

In your meeting(s) and or letter(s) (see below), don't give double messages. If you are not clear how you feel about something, such as being told exactly what is wrong even if it is very serious, then say you're not sure. But don't say you expect to be told if you're not sure you want to be.

Be organized. Express your most important concerns first, and be certain to make it clear from the beginning that this is a two-way street; you want to know the doctor's expectations, too. If you talk about prior experiences, tell the physician what did please you, as well as what didn't. The general tenor of the entire encounter should be assertive and positive, not complaining.

Emphasize to the physician that you understand your relationship is not a moment or a succession of moments. It is a continuing process. Every expectation cannot be secured at once. Acknowledge this. Emphasize that if the process works, you will become more and more willing

to assume responsibility. Most doctors will feel okay about "relinquishing" more and more power to people if approached in this way. It is also best, as you proceed, to indicate that you would eventually like to have an agreement (a better word than contract) defining what each of you can reasonably expect of the other.

Don't be discouraged if the doctor's response to your initial attempt to clarify expectations is not wildly positive or even negative. Whatever her reaction at the time, you can be sure that she will think more about the encounter with you. At some level of awareness and consciousness, your concerns will be acknowledged and processed. If, at the end of this first meeting (and remember, you can't reasonably expect more than 10–20 minutes), you feel that the doctor didn't "hear" a lot of what was important, ask if she would like to have anything repeated. It will be a good sign if she says yes. That will indicate a genuine receptiveness to what you are trying to accomplish. As part of this first interview, it is also important to ask certain questions which can help you predict whether certain expectations can be attained. Limit yourself to between two and four. If the questions are properly chosen, the *way* the physician answers them may tell you as much or more about him than *what* he answers. It is impossible to give you a full set of questions because they will depend on your particular expectations, but here are some, as well as the reasons for asking them, which have proven valuable to people.

1. What do you expect of your patients?
   The answer (and the manner in which it is delivered) should give you some clue as to the physician's humanistic attributes — a thoughtful, unhurried, non-stereotyped answer being more suggestive of genuine caring tendencies. It may also tell you

how she feels about partnerships with her patients.

2. How frequently do you refer patients to other physicians in non-emergency situations?

   You want a physician unafraid of admitting that he doesn't know everything, ready to acknowledge that and seek help when necessary. Therefore, what you are looking for here is not only numbers, or general tendencies like "a lot" or "not many," but some indication of such an attitude.

3. On the average day, how many patients do you have in the hospital?

   Unless her practice is huge, a primary care physician will not *average* many over three. Answers in the range of 6–15 suggest that the physician puts too many people in the hospital, and/or keeps them too long. It also tells that she is quite busy.

4. Do you have evening or Saturday office hours?

   A physician who schedules evening office hours almost always has some extra insight and caring into the difficulties of being a patient. He is seeing the world, to some extent, through the patient's eyes — a good sign!

5. What are your arrangements for evening and weekend coverage?

   What's important here is that the physician or her substitute, someone you know or know of, will respond to your call. Ask if substitutes will have access to your record (a big advantage of partnerships and groups). You will never know how satisfying the call arrangements are until you try them out. Asking others who have been patients in the practice for some time can also be *very* helpful. Beware of physicians who routinely utilize the local emergency room as a backup service.

6. What forms of medical insurance do you accept?

   Most physicians will *tell* you they accept any kind of insurance, but often this means (frequently with Blue Shield, for example) that they charge their usual fee (which is more than the insurance company allows), and you must pay the difference. It may be worth it, but it is good to know ahead of time!

7. How much time do you spend in the average week counseling your patients?

   Make it clear that you mean talking-listening counseling to provide information about medical decisions and medications, and to give emotional support and advice on family and personal problems. Perhaps this is something you don't need from your physician. You have found other ways to manage it — that's fine, don't ask this question. If you are interested, and the physician says yes, ask whether he makes special appointments or simply tries to work counseling into regular appointment spans. Again, the way this one is answered may be more important than what is said.

At this point, I wish to acknowledge that such meetings with your prospective physician can be difficult and sometimes frightening. This course of action is not suggested lightly. I do not minimize the various barriers that might keep you from carrying it out. It is, however, vitally important that you and your physician come to an appreciation of one another's expectations, and this is the best way I know of to do that.

THE LETTER ALTERNATIVE

If you are trying to revitalize an old relationship rather than start a new one, you may want to write a letter as an alternative approach or as a supplement to the one outlined above. Keep it to less than a page. Express the desire to clarify and reconcile expectations and to find effective methods of communicating. With some doctors, this may be a better alternative. They have time to digest your initial statement in private. However, if you choose this approach, always make it clear that you want to see them in person to discuss the contents of your letter. You might add what you think the goals for such a meeting might be.

NEGOTIATING AN AGREEMENT

Occasionally, with a receptive physician who has enough time, it is possible to actually negotiate an agreement in the first meeting. In most instances, however (whether the initial approach is by a meeting or a letter followed by a meeting), be ready to continue the discussion and negotiations later. Speak to the doctor again in a month or two. At that time, propose specific terms for an agreement. There need not be many terms, nor in great detail. They should include your most important expectations, clearly stated. The kind of statements found in the "checklist" in Chapter 17 usually suffice. Remember, coming to terms does not have to be done in person. It can be done by letter or phone. In many cases, a letter is better since your expectations will be in writing. However, at least one face-to-face exchange should have occurred before this agreement stage. A few additional pointers:

1. Use the word "agreement," not "contract." This will be more acceptable to your physician.
2. Be clear with yourself ahead of time about your points of compromise.
3. Phrase your terms as clear statements, not questions (e.g., "I expect a copy

of all lab results," *not* "Can you provide copies of the lab results?").
4. Make sure the physician clearly explains his expectations so that they can be modified if necessary.
5. Make it clear that you are accepting responsibility for your health and (with your doctor's help and advice) for your medical care as well.
6. State that if one of your high-priority expectations is in conflict with one of the doctor's, yours should take priority.

SUBSEQUENT STEPS

After the agreement is negotiated, you may need to review and strengthen your skills, identify an advocate, start a record, be clear about any medications you take, and think about yourself and your health. Other chapters provide many suggestions as to how to facilitate the diagnosis and management of your medical problems and acquire certain skills. Remember, also, that knowledge is power. It behooves you to learn about your medical conditions, particularly chronic ones, such as arthritis and high blood pressure, which you will be dealing with for a long time. Learn all that you can, and *want* to learn about them.

The task of finding a new physician and negotiating the kind of working agreement you would like to have is not easy. With time and attention to the suggestions made in this chapter, it can become a rewarding experience and prevent a lot of future frustrations and dissatisfaction. For some people the process itself has become a model for the subsequent relationship with their new doctor. Continued attention to the skills outlined in the last chapter and the suggestions made in the next one can enhance that partnership.

RESOURCES CHAPTER 18

Sagov, *The Active Patient's Guide to Better Medical Care* (Cited in Chapter 16).

19

The Office Visit, Being Your Own Specialist, Phoning the Doctor

THIS chapter will help you apply the principles and skills of Chapter 16 and 17 to three specific situations: maximizing the benefits of the office visit, being a specialist in the care of your chronic condition (diabetes, arthritis, heart problems, high blood pressure, etc.), and making phone calls to the doctor.

THE OFFICE VISIT

What can be done to maximize the benefits of an office visit? They fall under the general headings of preparation, when you are there, and feedback. The basic dimensions of the patient-doctor transaction (i.e., communication, expectations, and control and responsibility) remain the same (Chapters 15 & 16). And the skills of health partnership certainly need to be applied (Chapter 17).

Preparation

Consider taking a spouse/relative/friend (an advocate) with you (see Chapter 9 also). This is particularly helpful when you are in considerable pain, feel miserable, or are preoccupied in another way. Perhaps the comfort of his or her presence will be sufficient. But in case you are distracted in some way, brief the person ahead of time about your concerns and expectations.

Make a game plan ahead of time. Even under the best circumstances, time will be limited. Therefore, always be clear about your expectations, any questions you are likely to have, and how much you want to accomplish. In addition to the obvious ones like finding out what's wrong and agreeing on what to do about it, there may be expectations relating to how you expect to be treated and what information you want to be given. One universal expectation is that your questions be answered. It is so reasonable that it is often forgotten. Questions may include: What is the diagnosis of my problem? What is the medicine you prescribed? What side effects should I look for? Do I have to be concerned about other people catching this? Don't worry about thinking of all the questions ahead of time, but try!

Try to anticipate what will be expected of you. Forget about being "patient" and submissive. Your responsibilities revolve around giving information clearly and succinctly, being straightforward, and sharing any emotional or other problems that may have a bearing on your illness. Look at "Clearly describing problems or illness . . ." in Chapter 17. From that, you can predict the information the physician will want and be ready with your answers. You might even write some of them down.

If you think this will all be difficult, practice. If the usual patient-doctor relationship were, in fact, a collaborative partnership, you wouldn't have to practice. But most physicians still assume a superior position (consciously or unconsciously), so it is often difficult to be assertive and clear without practice.

When You Are There

Be assertive. Assertiveness has been discussed in the skills chapter (17). You don't have to deal with the doctor as though he or she were an opponent. Defensiveness is unnecessary. The business between you and the doctor is just that—a business transaction. It is important that you get true value. If you find that you are expected to be submissive or patient, you may have to find another physician, unless, of course, you enjoy or need that

kind of relationship; some people do.

Make your principal expectations clear when you arrive. If you are acutely ill, your most important expectations will have to do with getting better. If it is your first visit to this physician, it is reasonable to expect you will find out how the practice and the doctor work, and what is expected of you.

Ask to have information written down. This is especially useful if something sounds complicated or important to remember. If the physician doesn't have time to write information down, ask if the nurse can do it.

Ask questions when you don't understand. If the diagnosis (what is wrong), the recommended treatment, or anything else is not clear to you, say so, *no matter how elementary something seems.* It is much better to feel stupid than make a potentially serious mistake.

Evaluate the situation. If your top expectations are being met, there is no need to say anything. If, however, the visit deviates greatly from your game plan or is really going badly, you must speak up. "Doc, just a minute. This visit isn't turning out as profitably for me as I hoped it would. I'd like to get back on the track." Then proceed from there. Be firm, but not antagonistic. This may upset the doctor, but if it is asserted in an even tone, he or she is likely to pay attention.

Provide the physician and some of the staff, if appropriate, *with feedback* (see also next section). Give positive comments at the end of the visit if you can honestly do so. Nothing will reinforce the kind of behavior you want faster than clearly communicating that you are sincerely pleased.

Take your self-health record to the office. If you are there for a chronic problem in which self-care is basic and the doctor is essentially a consultant, this will greatly facilitate the visit. You can quickly show the doctor your progress since the last contact. If you ask questions, write the answers in your record before you leave the office.

Feedback

In addition to immediate feedback on a specific visit, regular long-term feedback is essential to improve the quality of your office visits. It can be done by letter, telephone, or during the same or a subsequent visit. It is rare for a patient to give a doctor feedback about his or her satisfaction. He may appreciate it a lot. It is also unusual for the physician to tell the patient how they are doing as a partner. Here are the kinds of feedback to give your physician.

- On his or her communication: is it clear, clean, and concise? Are your questions being answered? Are the answers adequate?
- Are your expectations being met? The first time you do feedback (and it is suggested that this be after a couple of visits, unless there is a very long interval between the first two visits), go through your list of high-priority expectations and let the physician know how she or he is doing; explain any discrepancies between your expectations and what is happening.
- Responsibility and control: are you participating in decisions to the extent you wish? Are you being given time to state your concerns? Is any information being withheld from you?

Encourage the physician to give you feedback. This may be unfamiliar and uncomfortable for the doctor, so be gently persistent. Emphasize that it is important for your progress as a collaborative partner. Ask if you are fulfilling the doctor's expectations, whether the physician wants any changes in the process or the relationship, and whether there are any specific points that need to be raised.

BEING A SPECIALIST IN THE CARE OF YOUR CHRONIC CONDITION

People with diabetes mellitus (sugar diabetes) who require insulin are routinely taught to give their own injections and regulate their dosage, change the amount and kind of food in their diets, take special care of their feet (because of frequent circulatory and infectious foot problems in diabetics), and diagnose and treat insulin overdosage. Diabetes is an excellent example of how physician and patient can collaborate in the treatment of a chronic disease. Mysteriously, it is uncommon for physicians to encourage patients with other chronic problems to participate in their own care to the same degree.

JAN'S STORY

Jan is 46 and since age 35 has had recurrent asthma, often extremely troublesome and unpleasant. During the first six years it got steadily worse, and she spent a lot of money and time with physicians trying to "be helped." By the fifth year she was taking rectal suppositories daily and two kinds of pills several times a day. The medication made her jumpy and irritable, and caused her heart to race much of the time; she still had to go to the local emergency room three or four times a year for injections of epinephrine to calm the attacks.

Five years ago, Jan was hospitalized for surgery on her knee. Soon after awakening from anesthesia she experienced a terrifying attack of asthma—the worst she had ever had. It was five days in intensive care before she could return to the general ward. She required steroid (cortisone) therapy for ten days. That, in turn, caused or contributed to an episode of psychosis, fortunately brief. Eventually it became clear that she had received a preoperative medication related chemically to one that she was known to be allergic to. She had told the anesthesiologist about this beforehand, but had not asked what medication she would be given. Even if she had, she probably would not have recognized the drug as dangerous.

Jan vowed not to put herself so completely in the hands of others ever again. *She would take responsibility for herself and participate in decisions about her medical care.* And she has. First, she learned about her medications, their potential benefits and dangers. In doing so, she learned a lot more about asthma itself and the circumstances that precipitated her attacks. She recognized many important substances to which she was allergic and identified the personal conflicts and frustrations that contributed to some of her more severe attacks. Then she learned how to deal with those emotional factors in other ways so they no longer cause or increase the severity of her attacks.

Now, she no longer takes medications on a regular basis, has not made an emergency room visit in two years, feels much better about herself, sees her physician much less frequently, and wants to tell the world about it.

Jan's story graphically illustrates how taking charge (changing from patient to person) can dramatically alter an individual's outlook and outcomes. It is also an example of someone becoming a *specialist in her own condition*, a vital part of Personal Health Competence. As an expert on your own condition, you are first and foremost a specialist on yourself. You perceive and report changes, learn ways to measure progress and improvement, and understand more clearly than anyone when things are not going well. You also learn the strategies that work for you in coping with limitations. Jan got to know herself and her asthma. She learned to treat herself; she gained control of *her* illness.

To be a specialist in your own condition, you do not need to learn all of the details about the disease involved. Understanding the variety and detail of a disease is obviously important for physician specialists who will see many different cases of the same problem with varying manifestations and responses to treatment. You need to be a specialist in your condition. The physician must be a specialist in the disease.

Being an expert on yourself is one of the most eloquent ways to be personally health competent. As I have said before, one can be ill in a healthy, competent way. The following steps will help you achieve such competence. They can be learned and used in any order; eventually, you may want to employ all of them. Many of the principles and particulars involved have been discussed in earlier sections of the book.

Acknowledge Ownership of Your Problem

Many people "don't do well" because they don't acknowledge the extent to which they are responsible for the problem. "It came from somewhere, and the doctor's going to fix it." Remember how Jan tried for years to have the doctor "fix it"? Fortunately or unfortunately, those who suffer from chronic conditions have a part in how and why it appeared. In any case, it is certainly *now* their problem, and they *can* do something about it if they take charge and use their own energy. Ownership helps them work effectively with their physician.

This can be difficult to accept. If someone is disabled by an accident that was clearly someone else's fault or has contracted a fatal disease of unknown cause, the inclination is to blame luck or (in the case of the accident) the other person, and shirk responsibility for helping maximize one's potential under the new circumstances.

It is important to distinguish between responsibility for what happened and responsibility for dealing with the outcomes. An injury may indeed be attributable to another person but what happens now is increasingly your responsibility. (See Beliefs, Chapter 17.)

David's story is an excellent example. For an extended period of time after losing his leg in an auto accident, David could only blame the other driver who had been seriously intoxicated for his plight. Later, through psychotherapy, he was able to accept responsibility for his *present* situation and accept the missing leg as a gift. Then he was able to move toward physical health again as well as progress in other parts of his life.

Grieve Your Prior Problemless State

One of the commonest reasons people with chronic illness have difficulty in "owning their problem" is that they have not grieved their prior "problemless state." What do I mean by this? Simply that whenever a large change takes place in a person's life, the prior condition (without the problem) must be grieved. Without grieving, the person can't accept and integrate what comes next. He or she needs to react (often with anger) to whatever the change is, accept it, say goodbye to it, let it go, and feel the sadness and grief of doing that. (See Chapter 10, Changing Habits.)

Decide How You Will Work With Your Physician and Become Skillful in Doing So

In working effectively with your physician, communication, expectations, and responsibility and control are the key. As always, defining expectations, prioritizing them, and being clear about your need to have them fulfilled is of first importance. To successfully manage a chronic condition requires that you exert control and responsibility the majority of the time. The collaborative partnership is ideal for this but it is possible to have a less equitable arrangement and still be effective as your own specialist (Chapter 16).

Many doctors have people with chronic disease see them too often. You may become so good at caring for yourself that physician contacts are rarely needed. Use your physician as a consultant. Know what your questions are; make sure they are clearly stated; write them down. And write the answers down when you get them.

Learn to Monitor Your Illness

If your condition needs regular follow-up measurements or tests not requiring complicated or expensive equipment, see if you can learn them yourself. If the doctor or nurse won't help you, try to find another way of learning them. It makes just as much sense for hypertensives to take their own blood pressure as it does for diabetics to check their urine. Measuring the mobility of joints is a monitoring step for arthritics and may provide added incentive for exercising those joints. Finally, don't forget to monitor the critical messages of your body: symptoms, feelings, emotional status, and energy level.

Keep a Record of Your Problem

Nothing can increase your effectiveness more as a "specialist" than keeping a record. A graph or tabular chart (flow sheet) as part of your self-health record (Chapter 4) is usually simplest (see Figure 19-1). Leave adequate space for monitoring observations (your self-awareness information, self-exam information, or both). If this is expressed in coded numbers, it doesn't take a wide column. Additional space should be provided for reactions and other events that may reflect a favorable or unfavorable change in the condition. With a little imagination, a lot of information can be recorded in a small space.

Inform Yourself About Your Problem

Use books, periodicals, other people, and whatever other sources are helpful. This can be fun. It can also, at times, be disturbing and scary. Despite this, most

FIGURE 19-1.

Date	Medication		Joint Pain						Stress	Other Comments
	ASA	Gold	A	K	H	S	E	W		
1/1–7	6	+	2/1	1/1	3/2	1/2	1/1	1/1	3–4	stomach feels okay
1/8–14	10		1/2	1/0	2/2	0/1	1/1	0/1	3–4	work difficult but going well
1/15–21	10		0/1	0/0	1/1	0/0	1/0	0/0	2–3	no redness in any joint
1/22–28	6		0/0	0/0	1/1	1/1	0/0	0/1	2–3	

ASA = aspirin, total number of tablets daily; gold — a plus sign indicates one injection. Joint pain is expressed on a predetermined scale of 1–4 for each set of joints, right/left: A = ankle, K = knee, H = hip, S = shoulder, E = elbow, W = wrist.

people find that the more they know about their condition, the more control they feel and the less fear they experience. (See Focused Knowledge Search, Chapter 5.)

Don't confine your reading to the general press and periodicals. Chances are that some of that information is wrong, particularly those pieces that relate to new ways of treating the condition — "miracle cures."

Of Course, You Can Never Know

If your reading turns up a new method of treatment which seems safe (your physician and non-physician advisors can help with that determination) and is not too costly, try it out carefully and see what happens. If it is helpful, continue; if not, stop. Be sure to enter the results in your record, so the information will be there where you can recall and use it easily.

PHONING THE DOCTOR (AND HER OFFICE)

Although enormous chunks of the world have no telephones, it is hard to imagine a system of medical care without them. In the U.S. the telephone is an invaluable adjunct to effective medical care. And it is important to use the phone effectively.

The purposes of phone calls are many. An obvious one is to make appointments. In every office a certain person handles appointments. If you know who that is you can ask for them and proceed. If the receptionist or nurse wants you to justify the appointment, cooperate. Tell them what they need to know and if they don't think your reasons are adequate, find out why, then proceed.

At an extreme is the call you make when you are so uncomfortable, worried, or in pain that you need assistance as soon as possible. Some receptionists are good at handling such calls, others not. The nurse may be asked to talk with you. Even if you are very ill you may have to be very assertive to talk directly with the physician. If you are feeling very uncomfortable, it is better to have your advocate get the doctor on the phone and then you can talk to her.

A common type of call occurs when you're not sure what's going on or what you should do. In both this situation and the previous one (if you are not too uncomfortable to think it through), try and prepare for the call as you would prepare for the office visit. Define your goals for the call and write them down. Write down any questions that you specifically want to have answered, and practice your opening sentence or two. If you are calling about a new problem, get the story straight in your mind so that you can present it clearly during the phone call. Plan not to take more than five minutes in all and less if possible — it will be appreciated.

Some doctors have special systems set

up for handling phone calls. In the commonest of such arrangements, the doctor will have a special time of day to answer phone calls. If you know what the system is perhaps you can postpone your call. If not, make sure you keep your line clear at the hour when he is expected to call back.

Finally, never hesitate to use the phone if you are deeply concerned or scared. If you can't get your physician or someone else at the office, call the emergency room or another doctor if you have one as a regular backup. On nights when your physician is not taking calls, try whatever arrangement has been set up. If it doesn't work well, be sure to let the doctor know the next opportunity you get.

Finally, a word about abuse of the phone. Some phone business will legitimately take more than five minutes. If you think it will, ask yourself if the matter can wait, and if so, just get an appointment. Otherwise notify the physician when you leave your message, or at the outset of your call, so that she'll not be surprised and irritated at the length of the call. It's amazing how much more patient people can be (doctors in particular) when they have some good idea of what the demand on them is going to be ahead of time.

For most people the physician's office is the main place they work with the doctor. It is important to make the most of each visit. This can be done preparing carefully ahead of time, following certain rules about good communication, clarity of expectations, and assertiveness while there, and providing and requesting feedback at appropriate times. When you have a chronic problem, becoming an expert in your condition is a rewarding and important experience. The guidelines for taking that kind of responsibility have been discussed. Finally some advice on phone calls to your doctor have been provided. A major issue in any contact with most physicians is the strong propensity to treat with drugs or surgery. The next chapter discusses that phenomenon and some alternatives to it.

RESOURCES CHAPTER 19

Begin with the *Merck Manual* or *Better Homes and Garden's Family Medical Guide* (see General Resources). Move to the library for general medical textbooks (you'll need to use the one which corresponds to the specialty within which your condition falls).

Many local hospitals have dial-in educational services where you phone in, ask for the tape on such and such and then listen. Such services are usually free.

20

Alternatives to Conventional Therapy: Why Not?

IN NORTH America pharmaceuticals (drugs) and surgery are the accepted way of resolving most medical problems. They can be highly effective, sometimes life-saving. In such instances their use is still compatible with the emerging age of alternatives and self-involvement. However, for some of the problems frequently treated with drugs or surgery, there are acceptable alternatives. While not always successful and certainly not always indicated, they can be quite effective when used judiciously. These acceptable alternatives are presented far too infrequently to the patient as explicit choices.

CHOICES: SOME EXAMPLES

To cure ankylosing spondylitis (a potentially crippling arthritic disease of the spine) you could take steroid medications. They might help the spondylitis but might also cause ulcers, high blood pressure, a fat face and thin bones. An alternative course of therapy as employed by Norman Cousins[1] might consist of high doses of vitamin C, faith, and funny movies.

For treatment of moderately elevated blood pressure, you can take pills. You may get good results. However, some of the pills will increase your chances of ulcer disease and could give you an allergic rash; others might cause dizzy spells, listlessness, and even reduction or loss of sexual desire and ability; alternatively you might try a low-salt diet, weight loss, regular exercise, and meditation.

1. Norman Cousins, *Anatomy of an Illness* (New York: Norton, 1979).

198

For many, this program will work well enough so that drugs are not necessary.

For undue work stress you could elect an exercise program or coaching in biofeedback techniques to help calm yourself periodically during the day. Or you might join the millions who take valium (the valiumaniacs) or other "minor" tranquilizers on a regular basis, exposing themselves to the risk of dependency, addiction, and dangerous interactions with alcohol or other drugs.

For torn internal ligaments in the knee you might elect surgery followed by several weeks in a cast and more on crutches, then lengthy rehabilitation. An alternative approach would be a program of exercise, whirlpool treatments, stretching, and muscle strengthening. This would probably require a longer recovery period and involve more risk of incomplete healing.

Larry made the latter choice.

LARRY'S STORY

One day on the beach, Larry turned to find his dog, Tawny, under vicious attack by two others. Ordinarily Larry is confident that Tawny will emerge unscathed from brief encounters but this time it appeared he might be a significant underdog. Springing to Tawny's aid, Larry stepped into an unseen sand hole and suffered a painful, tearing injury to his knee.

Examination showed that an internal ligament and cartilage of his knee was severely torn. Many orthopedic surgeons would have advised surgical repair within a few days, and Larry's physician cautioned that he might well need such therapy. Larry chose to try healing without surgery. It was a slow determined process, but with hot tub therapy, muscle conditioning exercises, and stretching, he returned to his regular running program six months after the injury.

Larry's choices worked although they were not what his doctor might have chosen for herself or other patients. You or I might also have chosen differently.

In any given instance there is often more than one choice. Many times there are other modes of therapy than pharmaceuticals and surgery. Awareness of this and a commitment to explore alternatives can give you a range of options that may (unless you have an unusual health care provider) otherwise remain hidden to you.

THE REFLEX APPROACH TO MEDICAL CARE

Medical care in the United States can be fairly characterized as reactive and reflexive. It is reactive because its predominant mode is to *respond to an existing patient complaint.* It does not help the consumer plan ahead to anticipate and prevent difficulties. The word "reflexive" is chosen to emphasize the "knee jerk" nature of how medicine reacts, which is usually by prescribing a medicine or surgery. The first thought of most doctors *and* patients is "treat it."

In 75 percent of all visits to physicians, the patient receives at least one prescription. The annual cost of these medicines exceeds $15,000,000,000. One in every seven patient hospital days in this country is the consequence of *untoward effects* of therapeutic medications. Untoward effects include troublesome side effects, toxicity, and errors (substitutions, too large a dose, too small a dose) in giving the medication. Out of the hospital, one in four prescriptions has some side effects, many of them serious. 5,000–20,000 people die as a result of toxicity or allergy to medications each year. The number of birth defects secondary to drugs is unknown.

The nature of some of the best selling medications is also relevant. Tagamet has proven highly effective in decreasing and modifying stomach secretions. It is highly effective for peptic ulcer disease. Long known as a disease of anxiety and tension, this condition is one classic model of psychosomatic illness.

Valium and librium are "minor tranquilizers." They are used extensively (6,000,000 new prescriptions each year for valium alone) for anxiety, nervousness, tension, and stress. Habituation and addiction to them is high and thought by some to exceed that to street drugs. While the cost in human function and well-being is not as dramatic as with hard drugs, it is, nevertheless, huge.

As a therapeutic measure, surgery is employed 25 million times a year in the U.S. and mostly under general anesthesia. The stakes are high. Surgery is costly, often dangerous, and can have serious effects. The average surgical experience requires about nine days in the hospital and more away from work. The cost to society is immense.

Of the 25 million major surgical procedures done annually in the U.S., it is variously estimated that from 2.4 to 3.0 million are unnecessary (*Confessions of a Medical Heretic*[2] says 90%). The 2.4 million figure is accompanied by a cost estimate of $4 billion and 12,000 lives. There are 400,000 tonsillectomies still done every year, 700,000 hysterectomies, 110,000 cases of breast removal and 170,000 of the newest high-volume procedure, coronary by-pass surgery. All four of these procedures must be held suspect in terms of efficacy when compared with doing either nothing, or something less risky, expensive, or mutilating.

Tonsillectomy is done almost routinely on seven-to-ten year olds in some communities. The procedure has definite value for people with repeated ear infections after two to three years of age and progressive hearing loss. Hysterectomy (the "bread and butter" operation of the OB-GYN specialist) is done for cancer

2. Mendelsohn, R. S. *Confessions of a Medical Heretic.* See Resources.

and other legitimate reasons, but an estimated 50 percent of the women in some studies reveals a normal uterus on pathological examination.

Radical breast surgery even for cancer may not, in many cases, be legitimate. For decades this mutilating operation was never systematically compared with less radical procedures in conjunction with radiation therapy or with radiation therapy alone. Now these studies are being done, and the less mutilating procedures seem to be just as effective.

170,000 cardiac by-pass operations were performed in 1982 in the U.S. The procedure still needs to be compared on a large scale with full "medical" treatment, i.e., optimal diet, regular exercise, weight loss, and appropriate drug therapy. Each operation costs approximately $30,000, *not* including time lost from work and recovery costs at home after discharge. There is a 4.5 billion dollar annual bill for this procedure alone!

Why does all this matter? If medications and surgery do the job, why not use them? First, they may not always do the job. Second, they may not always be the best treatment. Third, this knee-jerk approach to therapy subverts the process of self-determination and involvement, a prime tenet of Personal Health Competence. The "easy answer" is provided, and patient involvement is hindered.

This phenomenon — person presents a problem and doctor gives drug or recommends surgery — could not be so widespread without collusion between doctors and patients. Many physicians insist that everyone who steps into their office wants medications. Their patients "won't be happy" without drugs. "They'll go to another doctor." Many people tell you that their doctor "always" prescribes medicine. Both parties behave as though their own expectations had nothing to do with what occurs.

The same people who say their doctor prescribes for everything will often reflect concern about taking "too many pills." Not surprisingly a significant percentage of prescriptions are never filled. When they are, only a small minority are taken until they are gone. Proof is found in any family's medicine cabinet or around the house where there are 10–30 different bottles containing old and unfinished medications. Whatever their actual desire for a pill in the hand to deal with their problem, a lot of people really don't like them in their bodies.

Finally, thoughts on the universality of drug and surgical treatment would be incomplete without recalling the "placebo effect" discussed in the *mind-body* chapter. The issue is: how much of the therapeutic benefit occurs simply because the patient was convinced he would improve as a result of whatever was done? Alternative therapies (including doing nothing) can have similar impact if the health care provider imparts the power of her endorsement to the patient.

DOING NOTHING: AN OFTEN NEGLECTED AND VALUABLE ALTERNATIVE

The average person often denies or minimizes a problem for a time before seeking assistance. They may use home remedies or over the counter drugs or do nothing. Having decided to seek assistance, however, they expect to have something done—not nothing. However, doing nothing is highly appropriate in many situations, although seldom prescribed.

Doing nothing allows the natural evolution of a complex problem, which may provide the key to its solution. Doing nothing is also a good idea if there is not medication or a surgical procedure that will work. Most often it is a good idea because the precise nature of the problem is unknown. When this is the case, doctors and people tend to treat only the symptoms—the headache, cough, or nausea. This is called symptomatic therapy, and while not always a poor idea, it is practiced excessively. Take headache. Headache has numerous underlying causes. Some can be eliminated or ameliorated if they are discovered. However, we are conditioned to take aspirin or Tylenol without stopping to consider what may be causing it. With headaches, this practice seldom has serious consequences but it significantly decreases our potential understanding of the problem.

SOME USEFUL ALTERNATIVES

If alternative is defined as any treatment besides medications or surgery, there are a wide range of possibilities. In my opinion, various forms of exercise and body movement (including yoga), sound (but not trendy) nutrition, the meditative-relaxing activities, massage or other kinds of manipulation of the musculoskeletal system (including osteopathy and chiropractic), biofeedback, and imagery have the widest usefulness. Exercise, body movement, and nutrition have been the subject of previous chapters. The others in the list will be briefly outlined in the next section. Two commonly mentioned disciplines not discussed here are homeopathy and acupuncture.

Used properly many alternative methods of healing are more in harmony with natural healing processes than drugs and surgery. This notion of harmony or congruence is an important one. Later in this chapter, diet is discussed as an important alternative to medicinal laxatives for constipation. Changing what we eat is a more compatible or congruent way of dealing with constipation than using non-food substances.

Alternatives may also be congruent by providing certain basic needs that may not be met in the course of a hurried, materialistic living style. To the extent to which some alternatives provide them, like the touching inherent in massage, or the quiet, mind rest and solitude of meditation, they are congruent with health-giving, healing processes.

Relaxation and Meditation

A state of deep relaxation is subjectively therapeutic for people who are chronically stressed or feel pressured and driven. It can be specifically beneficial for people with high blood pressure and other stress-related problems (chronic fatigue, peptic ulcer disease, muscle tension with pain), as well as some assistance in reducing or stopping drug abuse, smoking, and heavy alcohol intake. Deep relaxation can be induced by transcendental and other kinds of meditation, the "relaxation response" described by Benson, autogenic training, progressive relaxation, and other techniques (see Resources). It also facilitates imagery (see below).

Yoga

The practice of integrating the mind and body is the essence of yoga. For the diligent practitioner, body and mind work together and upon each other to create a balanced, integrated functioning even in the face of disruptive internal and external stimuli. The aim of yoga is to help the body and mind maintain balance with one another or regain it as quickly as possible when it is lost. It is a method of cultivating and widening the range of man's power to adapt and adjust his internal environment in order to enjoy positive health and not just freedom from disease. Yoga believes this can be attained through the cultivation of good psychological attitudes, reconditioning the body to withstand greater stress and strain, and eating well and encouraging the natural processes of elimination.

Hatha yoga is the commonest form in this country. It is the systematic practice of a series of postures which increase flexibility of certain muscles (and, therefore, some related joints), strengthens the same or other muscles, and perfects balance. Although these physical effects are inevitable for anyone who practices faithfully and although yoga postures can be done solely as "athletics," many say that, "this is not yoga." Some adherents acclaim even more intensely the ways in which Yoga can be used to explore psychological limits and deepen one's spirituality.

Yoga is basically a way of life. Because of its underlying philosophy and its power to integrate the body's preparedness against both emotional and physical disease (a power, I believe, derived largely from steadfast adherence to the unity of body and mind), it is a general alternative of great value. It is the alternative to a non-yogic way of life; it is self-care of the highest and most integrated form; it is certainly a discipline through which one can attain Personal Health Competence.

Although only beginning to practice it, I am enthusiastic about Hatha yoga. I have resisted it until recently partly because it didn't feel good. I now know that some of it was not good for my body, my back in particular. In addition, I was hindered by a need to do everything well, which often meant excellent or better than someone else. By good fortune, I recently encountered a yoga expert of the Iyengar school with whom I took a short workshop. He reiterated again and again (in fact made a personal agreement with everyone in the class) that they could omit or terminate any posture they wished, particularly if it was painful for them. He was particularly attentive to the biomechanics of the low back and the large joints. He demonstrated with a miniature skeleton the proper alignment of the spine and other structures during various postures. He stated over and over again that we should be stretching muscle, not ligaments and tendons. He took special care to see that we were not bending the lower spine itself. Flexibility at the hips and of the upper spine produces the illusion of flexibility in the lower spine, but he taught that we should not try and bend the lumbar spine, either sideways, forward, or backward.

As a result of exposure to Sam I realize that yoga can be different than I thought. It can be just what I want to make it and just what I need if I advance slowly, move to the point of my own psychological and physical resistance, and then slowly on.

A note of caution, however. There are yoga instructors who are too enthusiastic, not just for people who already have structural abnormalities but for people who are normal as well. There are certain movements (e.g., back bends, the plow, the cobra, as most people do it) which can, through repetition, do serious damage to the low back. When you decide to do yoga, look for someone who will let you sense your own choice of postures and who agrees that you are the one to decide when to "come out" of any posture and that doing so will not be the occasion for ridicule. Most essential, find a teacher who does not insist that you work "through the pain" — or at least not until it's clear what that means. "Working through" the soreness of a muscle stretch is okay, but "working through" the pain of resistant (and essentially unstretchable) ligaments or tendons is something else. It is not always easy to tell the difference.

Biofeedback

A biofeedback technique monitors a particular biological function like blood pressure, and skin temperature, or muscle tension (with the electromyograph) and then feeds the information back to the subject's brain through some sensory mode, usually visual or auditory. The subject is instructed to try and change the function up or down. With proper coaching and the available biofeedback, he is then able to learn how to control the particular function. The coaching is critical. Some people can learn by themselves, but most will do much better with a good coach.

Take blood pressure. Most normal people and those with hypertension can learn to lower their blood pressure through biofeedback, although not all will be equally successful. Effective use of biofeedback as therapy for high blood pressure then depends on the person controlling blood pressure at times when she is not attached to the monitoring device. People who learn to take their own blood pressure have a powerful feedback tool. They can learn how various environmental and emotional factors as well as food and drink effect their blood pressure.

Biofeedback is also used to help people become skilled at total body relaxation, itself an alternative therapy. This can be measured indirectly through rises in skin temperature or muscle tension, both of which can be monitored with a variety of simple and sophisticated devices (see Resources). Self-regulation of the "pressured" feeling, familiar to many of us in relation to work, and the need to hurry are also subject to control through biofeedback.

Unfortunately the media and a segment of the public has had uncritical enthusiasm for many speculative applications of biofeedback. This has enabled exploitation of both medical and lay markets with equipment, sophisticated and simple, which may not have as wide application as that now projected by the press and some health industry enthusiasts.

Massage and Other Forms of Body Work

These alternatives are mainly thought of and used as means of treating disorders of the musculoskeletal system — postural abnormalities, rehabilitation after injury, chronic or repetitive types of muscular spasms, the neck and shoulder syndrome, low back pain (see Chapter 11). However, like yoga, they can, if properly administered and practiced, have significant psychological impact and effect change much greater than simply that of the condition under treatment.

Imagery

Imagery or fantasy is being used increasingly as an adjunct to other forms of therapy. In many centers it is being employed for diseases related to the immune system of the body (like cancer). It works best if total body relaxation is attained first. The images may be self-induced or "guided" by another person's voice. They may be straightforward ("imagine yourself completely well and engaging in one of your favorite activities") to highly abstract (like, "picture your white cells engulfing your cancer cells") to spiritually symbolic ("the area of pain or injury is surrounded by a healing blue incandescence").

Survival with widespread cancer can be significantly prolonged, occasionally with dramatic remission, for people engaging in a program of visualizing recovery combined with exercise and psychotherapy directed at overcoming resentments, goal setting, and coping with fear.

The process can also be used to assist in the management of other illness. The basic image sets employed by the afflicted person are (as paraphrased from the Simontons and Creighton[3]) as follows. First they picture the illness or discomfort in some manner that makes sense to them and then add to that picture any therapeutic methods that are being used and their effects. Second, the effects of therapy on the sick place or on improving the body's ability to heal are imagined. Then the body's own defenses are seen eliminating the source of the illness or discomfort. In the next set of images the person imagines being healthy and free of the problems and proceeding successfully toward their goals in life. The final set of pictures includes positive self-acknowledgment for taking part in their own recovery and (very important) imagining themselves repeating the relaxation-mental imagery exercise three times a day.

ALTERNATIVES FOR SOME COMMON SPECIFIC PROBLEMS

Various illustrations and examples of alternative therapies have appeared in other chapters of the book. In the next few pages three very common conditions (constipation, muscular aches and pains, and worry/anxiety/stress/tension) will be discussed in order to contrast some safe, generally very effective forms of therapy that can be used as alternatives to the pills usually prescribed by medical professionals.

Constipation

When I was a preschooler (before I had the courage to lie and give satisfactory reports), my mother and grandmother were preoccupied with my bowel function. When I didn't have a bowel movement each day (or if it was deficient in some characteristic felt to be important)

3. O.C. Simonton, S. Matthews-Simonton, and J.S. Creighton, *Getting Well Again*. (New York: Bantam Books, 1978).

their first tool was prunes. I never have liked prunes for that reason; they were used like medicine—"Eat them, they're good for you." And if I couldn't eat enough prunes to break the "blockage," then came an enema. That outcome was frequent enough that I vividly recall my mounting apprehension when I knew my bowels weren't "normal," the horror of the pronouncement, "Well, Peter, we're going to have to give you an enema!" I still can't abide prunes and prune juice, and enemas are non-alternative in my book!

In a large metropolitan chain-owned drug store, I recently counted 40 preparations allegedly useful for constipation.

The most prevalent causes of constipation are too much meat, not enough natural fiber, and too little exercise. So the main alternative to any of these medications is to change your diet. Decreasing the meat in your diet and eating more fibrous vegetables (carrots, lettuce, broccoli, many others) and whole grains (like whole wheat dark bread, oatmeal, granola), the problem can be resolved completely in most cases. Dried fruits (apricots, peaches, pears, figs, dates, raisins, and the notorious prune) are also valuable adjuncts. All of these foods work primarily by drawing more water into the bowel and providing more bulk to the stools. For most people they work better than medicine and they are "natural."

Muscular Aches and Pains

It is called "muscular tension" by the makers of Anacin. Commonest in the shoulders, neck, and upper back, muscular and musculoskeletal (including tendinous and fascial) pain can occur anywhere in the body as a result of injury (see Chapter 11) or emotional tension and upset. Some of my friends have at sometime or other described to me their own recurrent musculoskeletal

pain. As they speak, some of them unexpectedly make a connection between a specific kind of emotional tension and the pain. Others will do so as a consequence of my asking, "What else goes on for you at the times when you experience this pain?" Along with headaches, musculoskeletal pain is probably the commonest reason for using aspirin-like compounds.

The *alternative* therapy for this kind of discomfort involves relaxing the area (since a lot of the pain often comes from muscular spasm) and decreasing, rechanneling, or eliminating the emotional tension. Therefore, massage (which provides both emotional and muscular relaxation), gentle heating (increases blood flow), reducing or eliminating any trauma involved (which relieves both emotional tension and muscle tension), stretching, and pressure are used. Stretching counteracts the muscle spasm, which is really a constant, partly contracted state and allows the muscle to relax, thereby decreasing pain. Sometimes the maximum tenderness is in the muscle itself, sometimes in the tendon or fascial tissue that connects it to a bone. Often a single point in the tendon or fascia can be found that activates the entire muscle or muscle group into spasm. Somewhat mysteriously, pressure on that point can often break the cycle. It is a form of very localized massage called myo-fascial trigger point therapy. The body-work therapies discussed in Chapter 11 are other effective alternatives.

Stress, Anxiety, Worry, and Tension

Of the problems created by life-style, none is as widespread as this group. Stress is present all of the time. We need it to give motivation, encouragement, courage, challenge, and interest to our lives. When harnessed properly (like electricity which is channeled to run our factories and appliances, trains, etc.), it does that. But it can create pain, chaos, and disorganization when it is not transduced in a healthy way just as electricity can shock and kill when we touch the wrong wires. Tension is conscious awareness of poorly managed stress. Anxiety is fear which is poorly focused. Worry is the conscious obsession with unresolved problems or anticipation of specific events.

Muscle relaxants and minor tranquilizers work by suppressing neural activity, either in the brain itself, the spinal cord, or at the junction between nerves and muscles. They treat the symptom, not the cause. They often do reduce the severity of symptoms. We may feel better, and this often creates the illusion that we are getting better. Unfortunately, feeling better is not always getting better.

Alternative therapies include one group that can be done alone (exercise, relaxation techniques and meditation) and another set that requires reaching out to and being with others (an advocate, friend, or support group) in order to gain comfort, helpful processing, and support. Exercise and support have been discussed in other chapters. The choice of modalities is up to you. Different people find that different things work. However, for any really difficult or tenacious problem one support modality should always be included.

In and of themselves, drugs, and surgery are not excluded by the emerging health care pattern. There are many clear indications for the use of both. They are life-saving in some instances and provide effective cure or amelioration of many problems and relief of pain in many others. However, *the way* they are used and *the extent* of their use is counter to the new pattern. *The way* in which they are used (i.e., the knee-jerk response) minimizes patients' self-determination and involvement in their own care. The *extent* to which they are used excludes adequate consideration of available and effective alternatives that are often more congruent with what we know and understand about natural healing processes — physical, emotional, and spiritual.

The alternative of doing nothing is always important to consider. A number of others can be extremely helpful, both as substitutes for pills and surgery and as positive health-giving activities in their own right. It is often difficult to ask that alternatives be considered, but it is never a trivial or "crazy" request.

RESOURCES CHAPTER 20

Ardell, *High Level Wellness* (See General Resources).

Benson, H. with Klipper, M.Z. *The Relaxation Response.* New York: Avon, 1975.

Biofeedback Society of America, 4301 Owens St., Wheat Ridge, Co. 80030 (303) 422-8436. Can provide information about qualified practitioners near you and probably reasonable advice about equipment as well.

Danskin, D. and Crow, M. *Biofeedback: An Introduction and Guide.* Palo Alto: Mayfield Publishing Co., 1981.

Kustrubala, T. *The Joy of Running.* New York: Pocket Books, 1977.

Mendelsohn, R.S. *Confessions of a Medical Heretic.* New York: Warner Books, 1979. A very pessimistic but important view of what goes on in American medicine.

Pelletier. *Mind as Healer, Mind as Slayer* (Cited in Chapter 6).

Ryan and Travis. *Wellness Workbook* (See General Resources).

Sobel, D., ed. *Ways of Health.* San Diego: Harcourt, Brace, Jovanovich, 1979.

21

Being in the Hospital

"In the hospital you have rights but you are a prisoner. You are a bird with clipped wings, an animal in a cage. You lose all of your freedom, except as a consumer of medical care."
— A RECENTLY DISCHARGED PATIENT

IN THE hospital, people are invaded by needles, tubes, pills, X-ray machines, and physicians. Memories are probed and explored. People are seldom touched gently, embraced, or otherwise comforted. They are rarely talked to meaningfully by the people who live and work there. Much is unfamiliar: rooms that have not been seen, robed and masked figures that flit to and fro on unknown missions, and eerie sounds that unexpectedly penetrate the silent void. It is lonely; a sense of helplessness is virtually inescapable. Medicated patients may dream or lie awake as their fears and anxieties touch and grapple with the ghosts of the place. It is like a haunted house. Even for those who have never experienced a hospital themselves, the stories they have heard are much more likely to provoke fear than positive expectations. When is the last time you heard someone tell a pleasant story about a hospital? If you can remember, the odds are very high that it was from a woman or couple who just had a new baby!

THE PATIENT EXPERIENCE

In Chapter 15 I explained my objections to the word *patient*. Nowhere are those reservations more profoundly illustrated than in the hospital. Judging by their behavior, physicians and other hospital personnel much more often expect their clientele to be patient(s) than people.

On becoming a hospital patient, some or all of the following occur:

- In the admissions office, your name and basic information are fed into a computer by someone who may do his job like an automaton.
- You must sign consent forms which you may be too ill or frightened to read. Some fear they are signing away rights and privileges, as well as parts of their body.
- Soon after admission to the hospital (as in prison) clothes and other personal belongings are taken away. Your symbols of identity are replaced by a plastic band around the wrist or ankle, and you are clothed in that shroud of anonymity, the hospital gown!
- An endless series of seemingly endless waits take place, often in the admissions office, almost certainly in X-ray, for other special procedures, outside the operating room, and in bed.
- Loneliness and fear set in. You lie alone or in a room with strangers. You cannot see the nurses or their desk, or even tell where they are at any given moment. You are "connected" to them via a signal taped or pinned to the bed. The average doctor visits once a day, and his *busy*ness is never more evident than on hospital rounds. There is little chance to learn more than what the latest tests show. Time is not made for comfort and love. Many hospitals still limit visiting hours and visitors, particularly during the lonely nights, when they might be most appreciated and helpful. Loneliness and isolation are sometimes reinforced by seemingly senseless policy. A woman was recently admitted to a university hospital to be evaluated and treated for possible cancer. After two weeks her husband was admitted to the *same floor* for an entirely different problem. He was tak-

ing different medications than she. They were both confined to their rooms and asked repeatedly about and for one another. The hospital wouldn't let them stay in the same room because "we might get their medications mixed up."
- There is the provocation and strain of numerous assaults on your body: hard X-ray tables (for someone in significant pain, they can be torture racks), the drawing of blood, usually even more major and difficult experiences. You may be put to sleep or heavily drugged, while monstrous machines leer, click, and hum, often without explanation.
- You are relatively uninformed and feel choiceless. Even more than in the doctor's office, hospitals conspire to keep patients ignorant of their lab results and their progress. The next scheduled "test," medications and what they are for, and other explanations are often not forthcoming. Double and conflicting messages abound. Key personnel change every eight hours, and are often not the same from day to day, even on the same shift. Just when you think you have found someone to keep you comforted and well informed, he or she may disappear!
- Finally, you may be expected to understand everything perfectly, and endure without complaint. Sometimes it appears you exist for the pleasure of the staff, rather than they to serve you. You will be compliant!

These circumstances are not good for people, particularly sick people. They injure self-esteem and self-confidence and run counter to what we know about the body's recuperative powers. They impede and counteract the wonders people can do for themselves in becoming well. Recent evidence suggests that being a "good" patient in the hospital decreases one's chances of becoming well again. Instead of alleviating the dependence, loneliness, and vulnerability that almost always accompany illness or accident, hospitals operate to make them worse. Hospitals divest you of power, in this case the power to heal yourself.

HOW THIS PARADOX IS EXPLAINED

Why do hospitals and doctors permit circumstances that are counter to healing? Why such a price, in money and inhumanity, for the services which are provided? Some of my thoughts follow. They implicate the consumer/patients as well as the physicians and hospitals.

Hospitals are big business. In many communities of 100,000 or fewer inhabitants, hospitals are among the five largest businesses in the community. In smaller communities, they may be the largest single employer. Hospitals are run to make money. They are also a money-making work place for physicians. The design, equipment, and capabilities of hospitals are all developed primarily at the request of the physicians who practice there. The laboratory, X-ray room, surgical suite, and the procedures done in them are the financial life blood of the institution.

People are admitted to the hospital for serious conditions. They die much more frequently than those outside hospitals, and they are legitimately more limited. Therefore, a patient must consider at some level of awareness the possibility that he or she is destructible. The milieu, the appearance and behavior of other patients, the sense of urgency in certain areas of the hospital, all indicate that the hospital is associated with death and disability. Even if we "know" our condition is relatively insignificant, we are effected.

By necessity some of the work done in a hospital is assaultive and invasive. There is a great deal that is painful; a lot is unknown. This creates uneasiness and fear.

For many, the hospital feels paternalistic, foreboding, and powerful. It provokes the same reactions in people as a powerful parent, teacher, or physician did when they were children. If a patient's physician also produces this kind of reaction, there is double jeopardy, since the physician may be that person's most important contact in the hospital.

HOW ABOUT PATIENT'S RIGHTS?

Lately there has been considerable interest in patients' rights. The American Hospital Association, various patient-oriented groups, and other organizations have written and endorsed patients' rights. Like the Bill of Rights in the Constitution, "patients' rights" define important limits within which hospitals and doctors must work. They do not assure that a given hospital stay will be more pleasant, more caring, or less scary. A patient's expectations have more influence on the quality of the stay than any list of patients' rights.

Any hospital that is sensitive to your rights and tries to assure them will, in fact, be a better place to be than one that does not. But to overcome the real problems of waiting, depersonalization, loneliness and fear, expected compliance, ignorance, being uninformed and choicelessness, more is required. Success during a hospital stay depends on clarity of expectations, communication, and some sharing of control and responsibility between you and your doctor. In addition, it requires love and support from friends, family, your advocate, and the nursing staff.

SOME SUGGESTIONS

Neither the colors nor the mood of the picture painted above are cheerful; the hospital is not a place that helps one gain, or even maintain, psychological strength.

But you can alter this painting. The hospital does not need to be so grim; the hospice movement has shown that even dying does not have to be undignified or joyless. Being in the hospital may never be glorious, but it can be a growth experience. It can be gracious. You can use your skills and power to ensure more helpful and friendly care. The depersonalized, lonely, invasive, and mysterious nature of hospitalization can be minimized.

If you and your advocate prepare adequately before entering the hospital and follow through while there, it will better your experience. The suggestions below are directed at improving communications, clarifying expectations, and securing a favorable balance of control and responsibility and a medium of love. They are divided into two parts: what to do when *preparing* for hospitalization and what to do *once you are in* the hospital.

Preparing for the Hospital

This first group of strategies is for elective hospitalization, one that is scheduled days or weeks ahead and for which you have time to prepare.

Prepare yourself psychologically. Consider the kinds of experiences inherent in most hospitalizations as outlined on the previous pages. Think in advance about how to counteract them. Simply acknowledging that you may encounter all or some of these difficulties is extremely helpful. For example, it is reasonable that you will have to do some waiting. Imagine that happening and expect it. But it is unreasonable to be sent to X-ray and wait more than 30–40 minutes before your films are taken. Prepare yourself, if that happens, to clearly state that you will not tolerate a repeat performance.

Think about what you can do ahead of time to enhance or maintain commu-

nication. In the hospital, you must communicate with your physician, with nurses and other hospital staff. Sometimes communication with your doctor will be through the nursing staff. Try to get a list of orders your doctor will write so you will know in advance what is going on. Most physicians consider this a novel request, but it is a reasonable expectation that they provide such a list or read it to you over the phone.

Plan to take your Self-Health Record with you. If this proves unwieldy, at least take your Problem List. Clearly mark it "private and confidential." It will then only be available to those you choose. Also, take your medication list, as well as any medications you use regularly. This is extremely important. It will diminish the possibility of your becoming the one patient out of every seven that has an "untoward complication of drug administration" while in the hospital.

Ask friends and relatives to visit you in the hospital. It may be desirable to ask them to come at a particular time, allowing you to limit visitors at a given moment. It also gives you a chance to have them visit with you rather than having them visiting each other! Of course, you may just want people around you and not be bothered talking to them. In that case, group visiting may be fine. They can amuse each other while their presence and chatter comfort you. Make sure you warn all potential visitors that you're not sure how you'll feel or how much you'll want to chat with them, but that it will be supportive just to have them at the bedside for a time.

Get a commitment from a friend or relative to be your advocate while you are in the hospital. Get this commitment *in advance.* Even if you are entering the hospital for a relatively simple problem, *it is the single most useful preparation you can do.* The extent to which this person speaks for you and acts in your behalf will depend on how in touch with the world you remain during your hospital stay and how much autonomy you wish to relinquish.

A good advocate will serve as an extension of you and as an interpreter for you. He or she will not allow things to happen that you oppose. To be effective, you and your advocate must both know your reasons for being hospitalized, your expectations, your problems, the planned procedures, and, in the case of potentially life-threatening situations, your philosophy about extreme measures. To be a good advocate, someone need not be a close friend, but he or she needs to be clear on these basic matters (see Chapter 9).

Learn something about the quality of nursing care. The nursing care in a hospital is all important. If your doctor uses two (or more) hospitals and feels that the technical aspects of your care would be similar in both, then it is worth your while to compare the nursing care. Choose the one for which you get the best evidence that nurses *care* for patients. Care has several different meanings — serious attention, solicitude, time, affection. Good medical or nursing care will embody several of them. Ask friends who have been in the hospital about the attentiveness of the nurses, their concern for patients' comfort, ease, welfare, appetite, anxiety, fear, loneliness. This will take time but can make the difference between a miserable hospitalization and a tolerable one.

In the Hospital

The following suggestions are also written primarily for elective hospitalization, but many can be effectively used during an emergency or otherwise unexpected hospitalization.

Make your expectations clear as soon as possible. The most important expectations, for most people, focus on: (a) having enough time to talk to the doctors, nurses, and other personnel about what is happening; a busy doctor may want to delegate this to one or more nurses; this can work well if everyone understands what is happening; (b) how much you expect to be clearly informed (e.g., about all important results that emerge from the examinations and procedures); and (c) how involved you wish to be in decision making. Do you want to help decide about every test ordered and every change in management strategy or just major ones? If it is just the major ones, you and the doctor must define what "major" means.

It is important that such primary expectations be communicated to your doctor and the chief ward nurse soon after you are admitted. Don't be surprised if you have to repeat them after a few days!

During your first or second day, ask to see the patient services representative or hospital-based patient advocate. Most hospitals have such a person. When she or he comes, explain that you wanted to say hello and be assured that you could call again, if necessary, for help or assistance. Some of these agents only serve as advocates for financial matters, but many will be glad to help with communications problems or unfulfilled expectations as well.

Get to know the nurses in charge; find nurses who care. The nurses in charge of the various shifts may be the most important people you know during your hospital stay. Often it is possible to identify a nurse you like who becomes an important ally and source of information. This is like a gift when it occurs. But remember that all nurses have days off and that many nurses work part-time and must change shifts frequently. So, learn each day if your ally will be there the next one. Although disappointing to learn that your friend will be off-duty the next day, it is far better than setting yourself up for a day of frustration or feeling rejected.

Another consequence of rotating nursing assignments is variations in nursing styles. Nurses or nursing staffs will inform you and offer clinical interpretations to varying degrees. Even on very similar matters these differences can vary appreciably. If they do, don't be surprised. Say that you are uncertain or confused and try to get clarification. It is the obligation of the people caring for you to clear up any confusion you may have.

Ask to keep with you any personal items you like. Don't be intimidated by "hospital policy." If there is something that matters a lot to you, be persistent. If necessary, take the matter to the administrator of the hospital. This may sound like an unreasonable recommendation. However, it is an important way of combatting depersonalization. It is astounding how important a single article of clothing, a piece of jewelry, or even your own alarm clock can be in maintaining or strengthening your identity. It preserves that edge of uniqueness which differentiates you from all other people clothed in identical gowns, lying in identical beds, eating identical food, and often subjected to identically condescending care.

Ask permission, if you wish, to see your own chart. This may also be against "hospital policy," but if you are persistent, you will often overcome that hurdle. If you feel that the physicians and nurses are keeping you well informed, however, it may not be worth the trouble to argue about this one.

Wear your own clothes whenever possible. This is another way of combatting depersonalization. In some situations, there are real advantages to the traditional gown—people going to surgery, those who must have frequent attention to wounds and surgical dressings, and completely bedridden individuals who must use the bedpan. But for the majority of hospitalized people, insistence upon the gown is an outmoded, unnecessary regulation. Some doctors, nurses, and hospitals will still talk about cleanliness and contamination. But an article of clothing that has been unworn since last washed is extremely unlikely to cause any "break" in the hospital's cleanliness. In any case, it is well known that most in-hospital infections come from employees or hospital equipment and are stimulated by the abundant use of antibiotics that produce resistant bacterial strains. So, even if it is only possible to wear your own shirt or blouse, it is important to do so. Your body will feel far more familiar to you, and your morale will be better.

Find yourself a nurturing ally. If you're not comfortable doing this with an advocate or a friend, then pick out a nurse who seems warm, supportive, and nurturing. Whomever you choose, reach out to them, take their hand and tell them what you're feeling. Whatever that is, tell them. You must have someone be an extension of yourself, a comforting, warm source of helpful energy that you can depend on and turn to. Most physicians cannot or will not take the time to do this. It is certainly an avowed function of nurses and a reason that many people go into nursing. Hopefully you'll find a nurse who can do this for you. If not a registered nurse, try a practical nurse, an aide, or the person who cleans your room.

My friend, Sharon, hospitalized for cancer surgery needed to say, "I need you to care for me, please hold my hand, please sit with me for a while. I am frightened, this is a new environment, I need you to help me. Please care." This may be as open and vulnerable as you ever make yourself to a stranger but it is a matter of survival. When you need to cry, they can hug you. When you need to express your fear again, they can listen. When you need some trivial thing that will make all the difference to you (a wash cloth, more soap, a new tooth brush, your sleeping medication, a massage), they can help you get it or get it for you.

A huge part of taking care of yourself and of being competent and healthy is to let yourself depend on others when that is best for you. And in the hospital, for most people, it is best to have strong emotional support until you are feeling better, more secure, more "at home," less strange.

Most of the suggestions made in the preceding pages have a common purpose: increasing your control or at least assuring that your control is not diminished. You may not be able to follow all of them — you may not want to do so — but any one or more of them can be extremely helpful.

The suggestions can also be used to reveal your greatest fear about going to the hospital. Which of the suggestions offered is most likely to counter that fear? Then, if you are ever hospitalized, set out to apply it. You may find none that offer that promise. If so, sit down with a friend or family member who may some day be your advocate, and work out a strategy that does counter your fear.

Waiting, loneliness, fear, depersonalization, invasiveness, ignorance, and lack of choice — these are the scourges of hospitalization, not illness and disease. Find a strategy or suggestion that will combat the ones you find most upsetting and you will be more of yourself in the hospital. And you will heal faster.

RESOURCES CHAPTER 21

Ardell. *High Level Wellness* (See General Resources).

Sagov. *The Active Patient's Guide to Medical Care* (Cited in Chapter 16).

22

Your Journey, Your Health

THE perspectives and skills of health and well-being are more essential than any other body of knowledge. Yet most people do not behave as if this were so, and society provides no structured opportunity for us to learn those perspectives and skills in a unified, integrated way. This primer presents one person's concept of health and well-being, informed by many other writers and doers. It provides a framework on which anyone can build, modify, and change. It is not flashy; it is not the ultimate spaceship, but it is a solid and functional jetliner designed to specifications compatible with the present state of our art and knowledge.

In this, as in most books, the pathways and chapters are in linear sequence, one follows another. But such linearity is misleading because the pathways of health competence don't necessarily work best in sequence. They often work concurrently in the fabric of one's life. If I were a weaver or tailor I could have made you a tapestry or a garment in which the main themes interlocked and overlapped throughout the cloth. This would give a more accurate representation of Personal Health Competence than the linear chapters of this book.

So one way to visualize Personal Health Competence is as a fabric. The four pathways (Health Accounting and Information Gathering; Emotional-Spiritual Health; Eating, Moving, and Habits; Illness and Problem Care) are the main patterns in that fabric. The various perspectives and skills are the individual threads. The kind of garment or tapestry you fashion is up to you, but it will probably include at least parts of each main pattern, since they are all rich sources of health and work in a complementary way.

Another helpful metaphor for Personal Health Competence is that of a journey, your life journey perhaps. Like all journeys, it begins where you are now, lasts for as long as you keep moving, and has stopping places along the way. Like most journeys it can be fun, blasé, or miserable. Unlike most journeys it doesn't have to end. In fact as long as a person is working at being health competent, the journey will not end. In this metaphor the pathways are various trails leading away from the spot on which you stand at the moment. But unlike most auto trips, there is no best or correct way to go, and the only maps available are primitive. They provide guidelines but do not prescribe definite routines. Each individual may make unique and different choices. While you may choose to travel the paths in sequence, the journey is so magical it is possible to travel more than one pathway at a time. It may enrich the trip and make the stop-offs more delightful if you do. Imagine taking a trip across the United States. There are several routes to choose from and you might wish you could take them all. For the journey to Personal Health Competence you can!

Although you may progress along one pathway more rapidly than another or use only one for part of the journey, it may be important at various times to try them all. When you are chugging along one of them, again quite magically, travel on any other becomes easier. But there is no need to start them all at once or to be working on all of them at any one time. In fact, for some people, at certain times in their lives, one part of one pathway will be all they can handle. Others may concentrate on one pathway for a long time, like a dedicated artist or writer.

No matter which combinations and sequences you choose, there will be cul-de-sacs and dead ends. You will find places of astounding clarity, delicate beauty, and laughing laziness, and some frightening places as well. If your destination is clear when you begin, it may change as you progress or it may not be obvious until you have been traveling for a while. Everyday is a new opportunity. Every success, every joy, and every adversity provides substance with which to grow.

The making of this book has been an example of this; it is a metaphor for health competence in two important ways. First, it has evolved over time. It is much different now than when it was first "finished" three years ago, and even a lot different from when it was "finished" for the second time a year and a half ago. And already before the last corrections are made, before it is mailed to the publisher, and before I see the copy editor's work and the galley proofs, I want to change it again. But I know it is time to stop and evaluate. The evolution and elaboration of the ideas continues, but it is definitely time to rest.

Second, in the same way that any individual's particular pattern of health competence must enrich and reward them personally, this book has done that for me. Since I began writing several years ago, I have mostly enjoyed the task, particularly the struggle to bring the various chapters perceptibly closer to saying what I wanted to say in the way that I wanted to say it. Through that effort and enjoyment the work was definitely mine. I came to own it. But about a year ago I became additionally aware that more than anything else, the book was a vehicle for my personal growth, a way of fertilizing and planting my field, growing and harvesting a new crop all at once. Its purpose was to clarify my thinking, feelings, and spirit, to integrate certain parts of my life with the others, and to help me see certain interrelationships which I hadn't seen before. Most of all, its purpose was to give me an assessment of where I am in life.

And I couldn't have persevered without my own program of health competence. I encountered many disappointments before the book was ever accepted for publication. Frustration, tension, and a lot of hard work were standard for a long time. Occasionally I felt despair and anger about this marathon "pregnancy" and birth. My personal program of health competence helped me deal with all of those things—not always, to be sure, with calm or proficiency, but always enough to keep moving. My physical fitness, spiritual contacts, emotional processing, and intellectual curiosity have worked together to make the completion of this task a reality.

People ask, "What next? Where do we go from here?" I believe something comparable to Personal Health Competence can and will be taught in our schools. Starting in kindergarten or first grade and continuing through high school a curriculum of health competence could potentially provide everyone the opportunity to acquire competence in preserving and increasing their own health. Today, some pieces of Personal Health Competence are taught in some schools, but the integrated whole has not received a school or school system's attention. Whatever material is taught usually has more the flavor of *medical* competence than *health* competence. More is said about "what to do if such and so happens" than to reinforce the message that health is the greatest trip there is.

I believe everyone should have the opportunity to acquire health competence or some modification of it. Although other methods might work as well, my present notion is that a school-based, family-focused program of education and training makes the most sense. Programs should be initiated for faculty persons. Then those faculty members who become most involved in the work and struggles of attaining health competence for themselves can help the student learn. Such a program needs time and resources to succeed. One possible financing strategy is to make assessments on life and health insurance policies or on their premiums. If programs are run well, it wouldn't require a lot of money.

The orbit of Personal Health Competence can reach far beyond any one individual. As more and more people attain health competence and become involved in the struggle for their own health and well-being, their collective power speaks to those around them. In the sixties a small running club in Lansing, Michigan, and another in Topeka, Kansas, an army physician who systemized aerobics, and an American marathoner who bespoke health through the vehicle of the Olympic marathon together silently catalyzed the rebirth of physical fitness in the United States. Now, ten to fifteen percent of the country runs regularly or stays aerobically fit by other means. So it can be with the other elements of health competence, the emotional-spiritual components and those that pertain to diet and habits, and working with doctors. The world that each of us lives in can begin to resonate in harmony with the enhancements that you make or those that I make on the way to Personal Health Competence. And gradually the world of health competent people will become larger. The characteristics of anger and fear will be replaced by a base of love and peace. Someday a critical mass will be reached; the wave will crest and break and cascade brightly to shore. And we can all be riding it.

Despite its flaws, the world is fundamentally a good place; the people in it are basically good, not evil. That is my bias. Personal Health Competence has the potential for speaking to an audience greater than any one individual. As we each begin or forge ahead on the newest leg of a journey begun some time ago, the energy we create projects itself upon our world, and somewhere, at sometime in the future (five seconds, five years), we make an impact on someone else. All we must do is begin and sincerely engage in the process. Each of us who burns a candle can help light the world.

APPENDIX A

The Lifetime Health-Monitoring Plan of Breslow and Somers

THE following list of Health Goals and Professional services for ten developmental age groups is taken verbatim from "The Lifetime Health-Monitoring Plan" by Lester Breslow, M.D., and Ann Somers, published in the *New England Journal of Medicine 296:* pp. 601–608 (March 17), 1977.* Together with the suggestions made for periodic health monitoring in Chapter 3, they comprise the backbone of a health competent plan for periodic health monitoring. In addition, certain specific procedures may also be desirable for any given age group. Breslow and Somers discuss criteria for choosing these and give two possible examples. Those appropriate to your age group can be discussed with your physician.

GOALS AND PROFESSIONAL SERVICES

For each of the 10 age groups, a set of distinct health goals and professional services is desirable.

Pregnancy and Perinatal Period

Health goals:

1. To provide the mother a healthy, full-term pregnancy and rapid recovery after a normal delivery.
2. To facilitate the live birth of a normal baby, free of congenital or developmental damage.
3. To help both mother and father achieve the knowledge and capacity to provide for the physical, emotional, and social needs of the baby.

* Grateful acknowledgment is made to *New England Journal of Medicine*, Lester Breslow and Anne Somers, for permission to reprint the material from "The Lifetime Health-Monitoring Program" from the *New England Journal of Medicine* 296: 601–608 (March 17), 1977.

Professional services:

1. Prior education and appropriate counseling for parents expecting their first baby in physical, emotional and social aspects of childbearing and infant care, including family planning.
2. Antenatal and postnatal care for mother and baby, education/counseling for both parents, and risk assessment throughout the perinatal period, as needed.
3. Delivery services, including specialized perinatal care, as needed.

Infancy (First Year)

Health goals:

1. To establish immunity against specified infectious diseases.
2. To detect and prevent certain other diseases and problems before irreparable damage occurs.
3. To facilitate growth and development to the infant's optimal potential.
4. To provide a basis for lifetime emotional stability, especially through a loving relation with mother, father and other family members.

Professional services:

1. Before discharge from the hospital: tests for inherited metabolic and certain other congenital disorders; parent counseling.
2. Four post-discharge professional visits with the healthy infant during the year for observation, specified immunizations and parent counseling.

Preschool Child (One to Five Years)

Health goals:

1. To facilitate the child's optimal physical, emotional and social growth and development.
2. To begin the process of socialization through happy and effective family relations and gradual introduction to school and other facets of the outside world.

Professional services:

1. Two professional visits with the healthy child and mother (ideally, the father also) at two or three years and at school entry for compliance with immunization schedule, and for observation and counseling about nutrition, activity, vision, hearing, speech, dental health, accident prevention and general physical, emotional and social development.
2. For special high-risk groups, blood tests for anemia, lead poisoning and tuberculosis.

School Child (Six to 11 Years)

Health goals:

1. To facilitate the child's optimal physical/mental/emotional/social growth and development, including a positive self-image.
2. To establish healthy behavioral patterns for nutrition, exercise, study, recreation and family life, as a foundation for a healthy lifetime life-style.

Professional services:

1. Two professional visits with the healthy child (at six to seven and nine to 10 years of age), including one complete physical/mental/behavioral/social examination, with appropriate tests for, and follow-up observation of, any physical or mental impairment, including obesity, vision and hearing defects, muscular inco-ordination and learning disabilities, and completion of any necessary immunizations.
2. Mandatory school health education and individual counseling, as needed, for physical fitness, nutrition, exercise, study, accident prevention, sexual development and use of cigarettes, drugs and alcohol.
3. Annual dental examination and prophylaxis.

Adolescence (12 to 17 Years)

Health goals:

1. To continue optimal physical/mental/tional/social growth and development.
2. To reinforce healthy behavior patterns, and discourage negative ones, in physical fitness, nutrition, exercise, study, work, recreation, sex, individual relations, driving, smoking, alcohol and drugs, as

foundation for healthy lifetime lifestyle, including marriage, parenthood and career or job.

Professional services:

1. Mandatory school health education and individual counseling, as needed, for the above subjects, including a course in sex, marriage and family relations as a prerequisite to graduation from high school.
2. One professional visit with the healthy adolescent (at about 13 years of age) with attention to emotional status, vision and hearing, skin, blood pressure, blood cholesterol and contraception.
3. Annual dental examination and prophylaxis.

Young Adulthood (18 to 24 Years)

Health goals:

1. To facilitate transition from dependent adolescent to mature independent adulthood with maximum physical, mental and emotional resources.
2. To achieve useful employment and maximum capacity for a healthy marriage, parenthood, and social relations.

Professional services:

1. One professional visit with the healthy adult, including complete physical examination, tetanus booster if not received within 10 years, tests for syphilis, gonorrhea, malnutrition, cholesterol and hypertension, and medical and behavioral history. This visit may be provided upon entrance into college, the armed forces or first full-time job, but should be before marriage.
2. Health education and individual counseling, as needed, for nutrition, exercise, study, career, job, occupational hazards and problems, sex, contraception, marriage and family relations, alcohol, drugs, smoking and driving.
3. Dental examination and prophylaxis every two years.

Young Middle Age (25 to 39 Years)

Health goals:

1. To prolong the period of maximum physical energy and to develop full mental, emotional and social potential.
2. To anticipate and guard against the onset of chronic diseases through good health habits and early detection and treatment where effective.

Professional services:

1. Two professional visits with the healthy person — at about 30 and 35 — including tests for hypertension, anemia, cholesterol, cervical and breast cancer, and instruction in self-examination of breasts, skin, testes, neck and mouth.
2. Professional counseling regarding nutrition, exercise, smoking, alcohol, marital, parental and other aspects of health-related behavior and life-style.
3. Dental examination and prophylaxis every two years.

Older Middle Age (40 to 59 YEARS)

Health goals:

1. To prolong the period of maximum physical energy and optimum mental and social activity, including menopausal adjustment.
2. To detect as early as possible any of the major chronic diseases, including hypertension, heart disease, diabetes and cancer, as well as vision, hearing and dental impairments.

Professional services:

1. Four professional visits with the healthy person, once every five years — at about 40, 45, 50 and 55 — with complete physical examination and medical history, tests for specific chronic conditions, appropriate immunizations and counseling regarding changing nutritional needs, physical activities, occupational, sex, marital and parental problems and use of cigarettes, alcohol and drugs.
2. For those over 50, annual tests for hypertension, obesity and certain cancers.
3. Annual dental prophylaxis.

The Elderly (60 to 74 Years)

Health goals:

1. To prolong the period of optimum physical/mental/social activity.
2. To minimize handicapping and discomfort from onset of chronic conditions.
3. To prepare in advance for retirement.

Professional services:

1. Professional visits with the healthy adult at 60 years of age and every two years thereafter, including the same tests for chronic conditions as in older middle age, and professional counseling regarding changing life-style related to retirement, nutritional requirements, absence of children, possible loss of spouse and probable reduction in income as well as reduced physical resources.
2. Annual immunization against influenza (unless the person is allergic to vaccine).
3. Annual dental prophylaxis.
4. Periodic podiatry treatments as needed.

Old Age (75 Years and Over)

Health goals:

1. To prolong period of effective activity and ability to live independently, and to avoid institutionalization so far as possible.
2. To minimize inactivity and discomfort from chronic conditions.
3. When illness is terminal, to assure as little physical and mental distress as possible and to provide emotional support to patient and family.

Professional services:

1. Professional visit at least once a year, including complete physical examination, medical and behavioral history, and professional counseling regarding changing nutritional requirements, limitations on activity and mobility and living arrangements.
2. Annual immunization against influenza (unless the person is allergic to vaccine).
3. Periodic dental and podiatry treatments as needed.
4. For low-income and other persons not sick enough to be institutionalized but not well enough to cope entirely alone, counseling regarding sheltered housing, health visitors, home helps, day care and recreational centers, meals-on-wheels and other measures designed to help them remain in their own homes and as nearly independent as possible.
5. Professional assistance with family relations and preparations for death, if needed.

CRITERIA FOR INCLUDING SPECIFIC PROCEDURES

In deciding which specific procedures to recommend to implement the goals of LHMP, we applied eight criteria, derived in part from those adopted by the National Conference on Preventive Medicine, June, 1975, and in part from those used by Frame and Carlson: the procedure is appropriate to the health goals of the relevant age group (or groups) and is acceptable to the relevant population; the procedure is directed to primary or secondary prevention of a clearly identified disease or condition that has a definite effect on the length or quality of life; the natural history of the disease (or diseases) associated with the condition is understood sufficiently to justify the procedure as outweighing any adverse effects of intervention; for purposes of screening, the disease or condition has an asymptomatic period during which detection and treatment can substantially reduce morbidity or mortality or both; acceptable methods of effective treatment are available for conditions discovered; the prevalence and seriousness of the disease or condition justify the cost of intervention; the procedure is relatively easy to administer, preferably by paramedical personnel with guidance and interpretation by physicians, and generally available at reasonable cost; and resources are generally available for follow-up diagnostic or therapeutic intervention if required.

As noted in the Report of Task Force III, National Conference on Preventive Medicine:

In deciding upon incorporation of preventive medical procedures into personal health services, i.e., in applying the criteria, "prudence" becomes a major factor. The evidence available for decision is usually imperfect. Scientific skepticism is properly applicable not only toward many things that have been included in medicine for years but also toward what is new in preventive medicine.

One reason for continuing uncertainty in the minds of some experts about the value of certain procedures and the necessity of relying on judgement rather than overwhelming scientific evidence, is that we do not have the means, traditions, or system for rationally examining in desirable detail everything that is done or proposed in medicine. . . .

Steps toward improving this situation are underway in the form of clinical trials in general medicine and mass trials in preventive medicine. . . . Meanwhile, because such trials may require years to complete and even then may not be definitive, and because for other procedures in preventive medicine such trials are not feasible, it will be necessary to make some decisions on the basis of "prudent" evaluation of what evidence exists.

The emphasis on "prudence" in the above quotation makes explicit what is common and necessary in medicine as a whole—namely, taking some action based on judgment of an admittedly incomplete set of facts.

SPECIFIC PROCEDURES FOR TWO AGE GROUPS

Applying these criteria to two of the age groups discussed above, *Infancy* and *Older Middle Age*, we suggest the following list of specific procedures. The first was relatively easy to draw up. The basic criteria for well-baby care are fairly well established in both private practice and public-health clinics.

Infancy (First Year)

Specific screening procedures to be carried out before discharge from the hospital or during four post-discharge visits are as follows:

Older Middle Age (40 to 59 Years)

By contrast with the list for infants, it is impossible at present to list for this age group preventive procedures that would receive universal professional approval. The spectrum of opinion still varies from those who hold firmly to the need for a complete annual "checkup" to those who claim that nearly all preventive services are wasted.

The following list—featuring one complete professional examination at 40 and subsequent examinations at five-year intervals, with a few selected tests, which could generally be handled by nonphysician personnel, at intervals of two to three years (i.e., once between the five-year intervals)—is a compromise. It is based on the criteria set forth above and reflects our judgment of carefully evaluated experience to date.

Note, particularly, the absence of x-ray examination of the lungs and tonometry as routine screening procedures. Except for heavy smokers and other high-risk groups, the routine chest x-ray study can no longer be justified at this age. For glaucoma, both the reliability of the existing screening procedures and the value of treatment before the onset of visual field loss are now being questioned.

Among other tests whose routine application is professionally questioned by some are those for diabetes. The standard tests—fasting blood sugar and abnormal glucose tolerance—are reasonably reliable, but the value of detecting the disease in the asymptomatic stage in this age group, as compared to withholding treatment until symptoms appear, is not clear. The importance of detecting breast cancer as early as possible is generally recognized. However, there is no good evidence, as yet, that mammography contributes to that purpose among women under 50.

Suspected or Possible Condition	*Procedure*
Metabolic disorders	Phenylketonuria screening
Gonorrheal ophthalmia	Silver nitrate prophylaxis
Diphtheria, tetanus & pertussis Measles, mumps, rubella } Poliomyelitis	Immunization
Bleeding due to hypoprothrombinemia	Prophylactic administration of vitamin K
Anemia	Hematocrit

Growth and development disorders,
    including congenital dislocation of hip
	Developmental assessment, including
	    observation for congenital disorders,
	    height & weight

On the other hand, there is strong emphasis on self-monitoring. Patient responsibility in this respect, however, can be increased by periodic reports to, and instructions from, a physician or other qualified health professional.

Specific screening procedures are to be carried out as follows:

Suspected or Possible Condition	Screening Procedure
Intervals of 2–3 years	
Malnutrition, including obesity	Weight & height measurements — history of nutrition & activity*
Hypertension & associated conditions	Blood pressure*
Cervical cancer	Papanicolaou smear
Intestinal cancer	Stool for blood*
Breast cancer	Professional breast examination, with mammography for those >50*
Complications from smoking	Smoking history
Endometrial cancer (postmenopausal women)	History of postmenopausal bleeding*

*Once /yr > 50.

5-yr intervals	
Coronary-artery disease	Cholesterol, triglycerides, electrocardiography
Alcoholism	Drinking history
Anemia	Hematocrit
Diabetes	Blood sugar test (fasting & 1-hr. p.c. suggested)
Vision defect	Refraction
Hearing defect	Audiogram

High-risk groups	
Add to 5-yr. Intervals:	
Tuberculosis	PPD [skin test]
Syphilis	VDRL [blood test]

APPENDIX B

Status of Various States on Patient Access to Medical Records

THE states shown in Table 1 explicitly provide patients access to their records by statute or case law. If a state is not listed here there was either no legislation (as of 1980) or the only legislation related to mental health cases (see Medical Records: Getting Yours in Chapter 4 for more details).[1]

1. Grateful acknowledgment is made to the Heath Research Group, publishers of *Medical Records: Getting Yours*, for permission to utilize the data in Appendix B which is abstracted and rearranged from a chart in that book entitled "A State by State Survey of Laws," pp. 34–42.

TABLE 1. States That Explicitly Provide Patient Access to Their Records by Statute or Case Law

State	Kind of Records		Kind of Access		Indirect Access
State	*Phys.*	*Hosp.*	*Inspect*	*Copy*	*Only*
Alabama	X	X	X	X	
California	X	X			X
Colorado*	X	X	X	X	
Connecticut		X	X	X	
Florida*	X	X	X[1]	X	
Hawaii	X	X		X	
Illinois*	X	X	X	X[1]	X[1a]
Indiana		X[2]	X[2]	X[2]	
Louisiana	X[3]	X[3]		X[3]	X
Maine		X		X	
Massachusetts*		X	X	X	
Michigan	X	X	X		
Minnesota	X	X			X
Mississippi		X			X
Nebraska		X	X	X	
Nevada	X	X	X	X	
New Jersey		X	X		
New York	X			X	
Ohio		X			
Oklahoma*	X	X	X	X	
Oregon*	X	X		X	
South Dakota		X		X	
Tennessee		X			X
Texas		X			
Utah	X	X			X
Virginia	X	X	X[4]	X[4]	

1. Applies to hospital records only.
1a. Applies to doctor's records only.
2. A statute provides only that hospital records should be "readily available to the patient."
3. A statute provides for direct access in the specific situation where medical information has been transmitted to a third person.
4. The right to inspect records refers to official records only. The right to copy records applies only in the context of a lawsuit.

In the states in Table 1, you should be able to acquire your records as indicated (or summaries of them) without legal difficulty, although perhaps not without red tape. Most states will require authorization and payment of copying costs. Some may not release the records until after discharge from the hospital. Some qualify access by saying it is okay unless "detrimental to health of patient."

* Those states indicated by an asterisk may exclude psychiatric and/or psychological summaries (which would probably be obtainable by court order).

APPENDIX C

One Dependable Flexibility and Muscle Balance Routine

THIS routine involves attending explicitly to each of the following groups of muscles and their related joints: neck, shoulders and arms, low back and buttocks, abdomen, front of the legs, and the back of the legs. *Remember to breathe regularly during all stretches while concentrating your attention on the muscles being stretched.*

NECK

Stretching the neck should be done while standing or sitting erect. Neck stretches can be shorter in duration than others because the muscles are shorter and less powerful. The head is moved so that one ear comes as close as possible to the corresponding shoulder. This stretches the opposite side of the neck. The head is then moved in a similar manner to the other side. After that stretch, move it forward so that your chin touches the chest. Then gently back until the front skin of the neck is taut. You may feel clicking sensations in the spine of the neck during these movements; this is okay. If you feel pain in the neck or arms, do not continue. If there is tightness which is not taken care of by these four movements, then incline the head forward at a 45-degree angle on each side, chin toward the breast nipple, holding that position until the tightness subsides. (See Figure C-1) Always return the head to the neutral

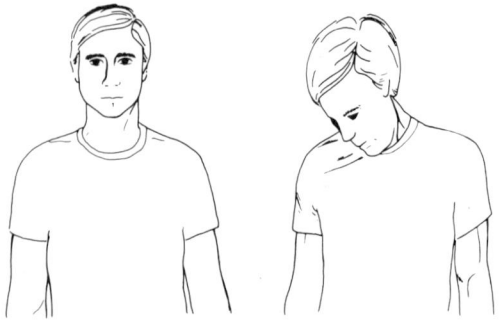

FIGURE C-1.

226

position before beginning the next stretch. *Do not rotate the head through circles.* This will damage the small joints of the neck if done repeatedly over months or years. Do only the six movements — to the shoulders on either side, to the front, to the back, and to the front at 45 degrees on each side.

Arms and Shoulders

The following exercises for flexibility of the arms and shoulders are a combination of stretching and loosening movements. As in the neck, the 30–60 second time requirements do not apply. The movements are repetitive. They are all done standing erect with your feet shoulder width apart and knees straight or slightly bent but not locked.

1. With arms stretched out to the sides from the shoulders, rotate them in 16-inch circles while keeping them straight. Do this ten times in each direction. (See Figure C-2.)

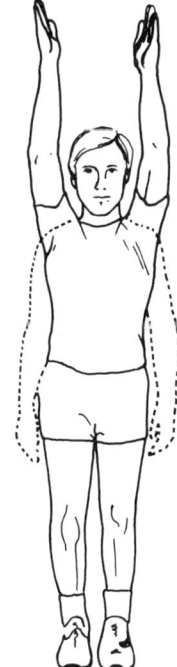

FIGURE C-3.

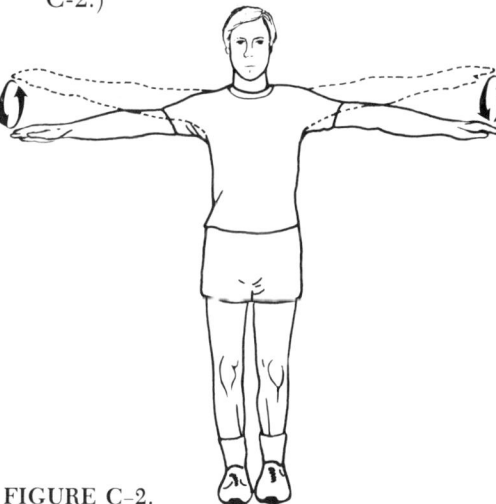

FIGURE C-2.

2. With arms at sides, lift them until they meet over your head, stretch them upwards for ten seconds, and return them to your sides. Repeat ten times. (See Figure C-3.)

3. Starting with your arms above your head (but not together) and keeping them parallel, swing them forward and down beside your legs, and then behind you. Hold for a few seconds, then return them to the starting position. Repeat this ten times as well. (See Figure C-4.)

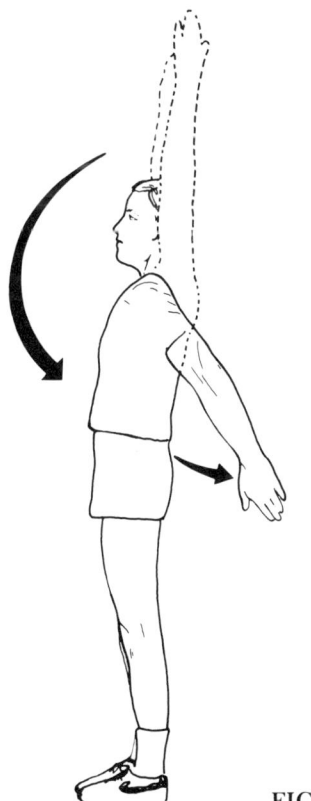

FIGURE C-4.

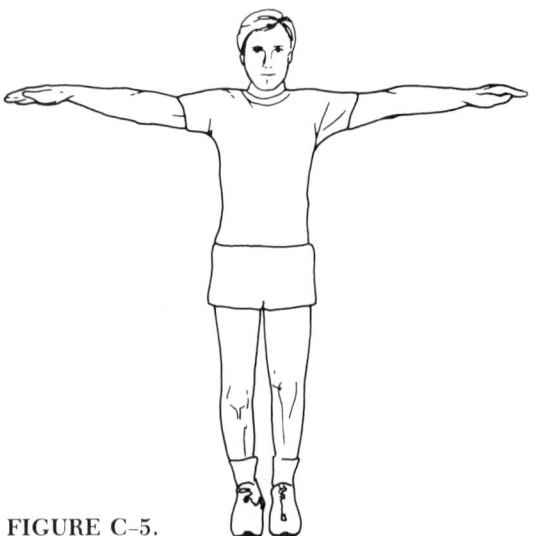

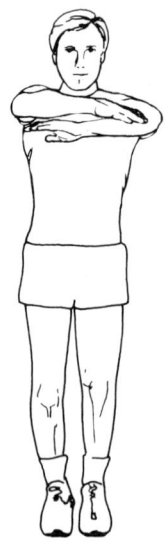
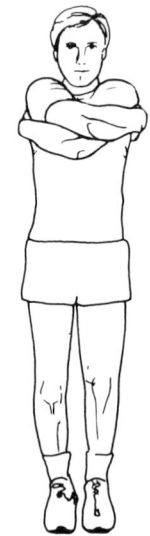

FIGURE C-5.

4. Again beginning with the arms stretched out to your sides (as in 1), cross them in front of your chest, stretch them briefly and then return. Repeat this ten times. (See Figure C-5.)

LOW BACK AND BUTTOCKS

These exercises are done on the floor or soft ground. A mat or carpet is desirable.

1. Lying on your back, knees bent, feet flat on the floor, force the small of your back downward into the surface and hold for 15–20 seconds. (See Figure C-6.) Breathe.

FIGURE C-6.

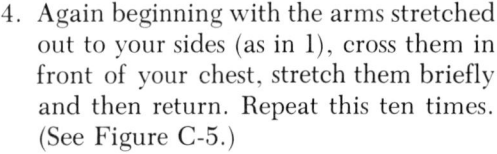

If this is being done correctly, you will not be able to get your hand between the small of your back and the floor or ground. It is sometimes called a pelvic tilt because the pelvis actually rotates forward slightly (toward the front of your body) to accomplish the straightening of the spine. Repeat three times.
2. Now straighten both legs and then raise the left leg, while bending it at the knee so that you can hook your left elbow around that knee and hold the upper calf in your left hand. Grab your left foot with

the right hand. Apply steady pressure on the leg toward your head and slightly away from your body, as though you were trying to put your foot behind your head. (See Figure C-7.) You should feel stretching in your buttock. Hold for a major stretch. Breathe! After relaxing the stretch but before releasing your hold on the leg, roll onto your right side and then do the stretch again. This stretches a slightly different part of the buttock. Repeat the entire procedure with the other leg.

FIGURE C-7.

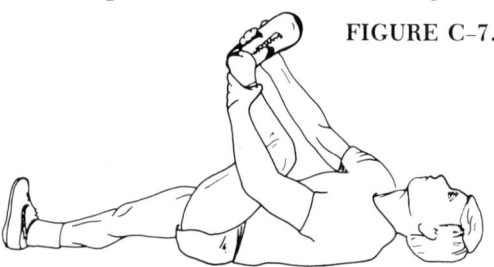

3. Still on your back, bring both knees toward your chest and clasp them with your hands or forearms. Pull them firmly to-

FIGURE C-8.

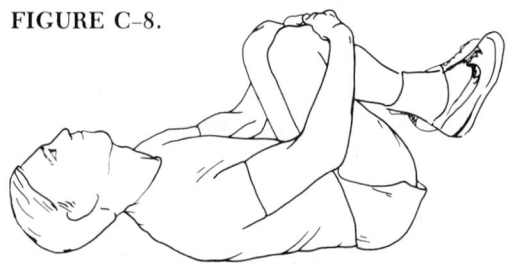

ward your chest making sure that the lower part of your spine does not leave the floor. (See Figure C-8.) Try pushing your tailbone and the back of your buttocks away from your trunk. Hold 15–20 seconds. Breathe regularly all the time.

4. Rolling on to your stomach, rest your head comfortably on your hands. Relax your arms. Now lift the right leg off the floor as far as you comfortably can with the knee straight but not locked. Hold a few seconds, then return to floor. Repeat ten times. Do the same with the other leg. (See Figure C-9.)

FIGURE C–9.

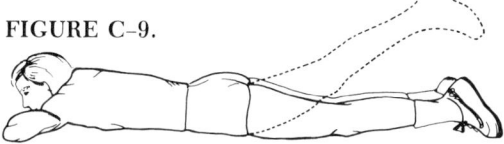

ABDOMEN

These can be done during the low back/buttocks series before turning on your stomach.

1. The basic exercise here is called an abdominal curl. It is the little brother of the full sit-up but is equally effective for strengthening the abdominal muscles and is not potentially damaging to the lower spine. It is done as in Figure C-10 but with hands on the chest.

2. If your abdomen is already in good tone, these may be too easy. In that case, merely clasp your hands behind your neck and do the same exercise. (See Figure C-10.)

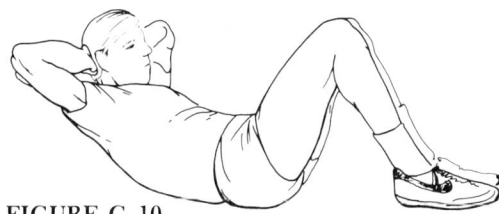

FIGURE C–10.

3. To give more attention to the side muscles in the abdominal wall, do the same basic exercise as in #2, but touch your right elbow to the left knee. The foot leaves the floor and you bring the knee back while moving the elbow forward. This provides slight twist to the thoracic spine and uses slightly different abdominal muscle groups than the previous exercise. Hold the contact for two seconds then return to the resting position and repeat with the opposite elbow and knee. (See Figure C-11.) Do the complete sequence five times to start.

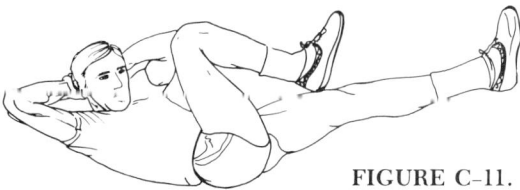

FIGURE C–11.

FRONT OF EACH LEG

The quadriceps are the large muscles grouped on the front of the thigh. To strengthen these for good balance around the knee joint, climb stairs or hills a couple times a week, either as part of your regular exercise program or at some other time. Four or five flights of stairs repeated three or four times is a good starter for most people. Be careful — use your judgment. To stretch this muscle group, stand balanced with feet shoulder width apart. While steadying yourself with the left hand on a wall or chair, bend the right lower leg up behind you and grab the ankle with your right hand. Straighten your body so that you are erect. Then move the knee and thigh back, and you should feel stretching in the quadriceps. Be careful not to pull foot into buttock. (See Figure C-12.) Hold for a major stretch. Repeat on the other side. If you can learn to do this without support, it is excellent for posture and body balance.

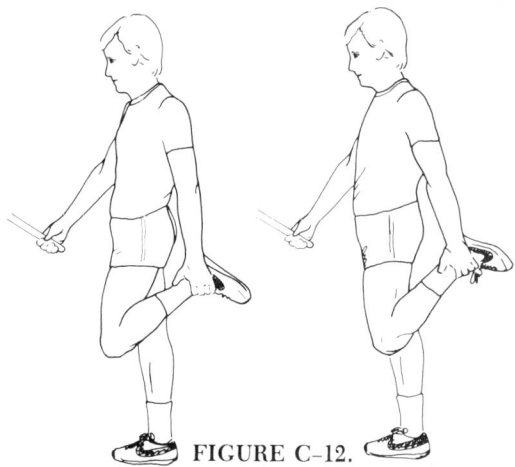

FIGURE C–12.

BACK OF EACH LEG

The upper part (back of the thigh or hamstring) and the lower part (calf or gastrocnemius) must be stretched separately.

For the Calf

1. Stand on a step where you can balance yourself by placing a hand on the railing. Place the ball of the right foot on the edge of the step so that somewhat more than the back half of the foot hangs over the edge of the step. Keeping the right knee straight but not locked, *gradually* transfer all or most of your weight onto the ball of the right foot. This will stretch the right calf. (See Figure C-13.) This is a major

FIGURE C–13.

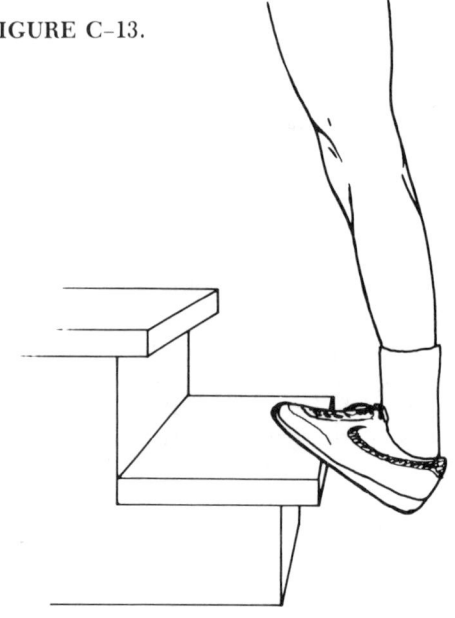

stretch. Before moving to the other foot bend the knee slightly — this stretches the lower part of the muscle belly. Do the other foot in the same way. It is also helpful at times to do the complete stretch as described, then repeat it with the heel a few inches to the right, and again with the heel a few inches to the left.
2. Place both hands against a wall at shoulder level. Keeping arms straight place the left foot on the floor under your chest. Extend the right leg back approximately three or four feet behind the other one (depending on your height and flexibil-

FIGURE C–14.

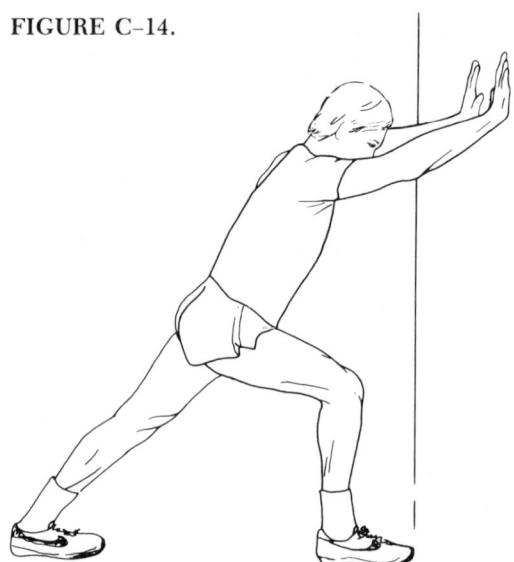

ity). Both feet should point straight at the wall. Keeping the arms straight push onto the back foot so that the heel reaches or gets closer to the floor. Keep the knee of the back leg straight, feel the stretch in the calf. (See Figure C-14.) Major stretch. Repeat with the knee slightly bent. Do the same with the legs reversed.

For the Thigh

1. While on your back for other exercises, get a five–six-foot length of rope or a band of cloth and put it around the ball of your foot so that you are holding one end of it in each hand (See Figure C-15). Keeping the other leg flat on the floor and the knee of the active leg straight (but not tightly locked), bring the rope back so that the stretch is felt in the thigh and buttock (and sometimes the calf as well). Breathe deeply and slowly and with each expiration pull back slightly further on the tie. (See Figure C-15.) Major stretch.

FIGURE C–15.

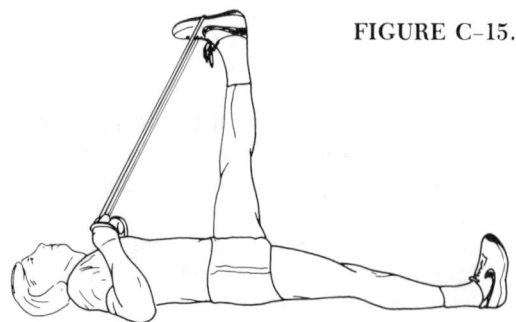

2. Standing erect with big toes together and heels an inch or so apart, place hands on hips. Keeping knees straight (not locked), bend forward from the pelvis keeping upper back straight; do not round the back. The objective is to end up with the upper body horizontal to the floor or as close to that as you can get, face looking directly at the floor. You will feel the stretch in your hamstrings (back of thigh) and perhaps the gastrocnemius (back of calf) as well. (See Figure C-16.) Major stretch. You will see that this is related to the old lean-over-and-touch-your-toes routine. That one is very bad for the lower back. In this stretch, the pelvis rotates forward from the hips but the lower back does not bend.

3. Find a bench, table, or sturdy chair back that is about the level of your waist. Standing flat on one foot, place the other heel on the surface of the bench or table or the back of the chair. Do not bend forward from the waist. The stretch can be obtained by straightening the knee then forcing your torso slightly forward while keeping it erect or almost erect. (See Figure C-17.) Major stretch. This is a variation on the "hurdle stretch" in which you also bend forward onto the extended leg. Unless you are practicing yoga and have no trouble with your back, do not bend forward. It too has the potential for injuring your back, and the back of the thigh can be stretched just as well without bending forward.

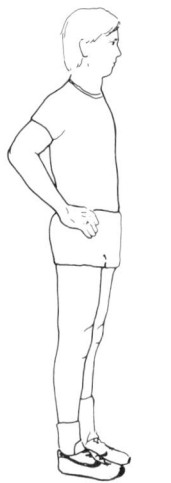
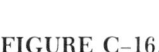
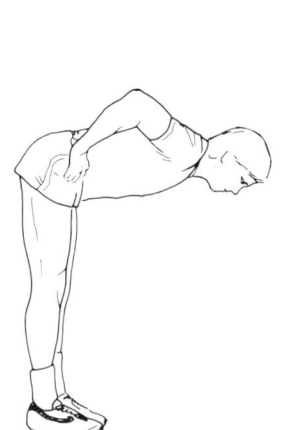

FIGURE C–16.

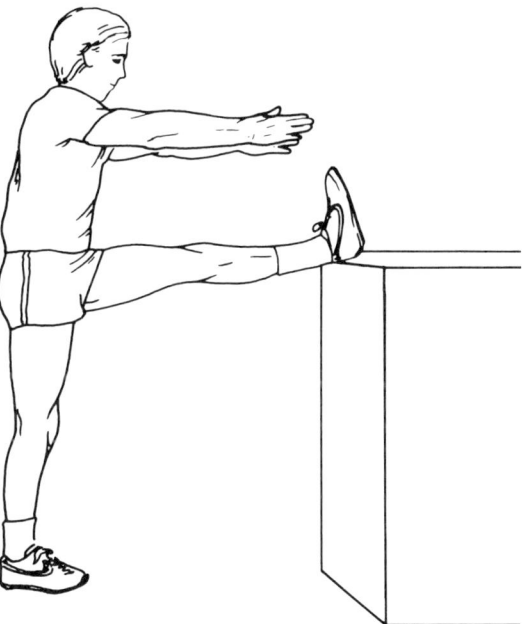

FIGURE C–17.

General Resources

THE following resources provide information and other types of assistance as indicated. The emphasis in this list is on matters of health and well-being but some sources deal with medical problems as well.

BOOKS AND PERIODICALS

1. *American Health: Fitness of Body and Mind*, P.O. Box 10035, Des Moines, Iowa 50340.

   A newer periodical that focuses somewhat more on illness than Medical Self Care but maintains good balance. Published bimonthly. On most newstands.

2. Ardell, D. *High Level Wellness, An Alternative to Doctors, Drugs and Disease*. Emmaus, PA: Rodale Press, 1977.

   One of the basic books on the wellness idea and movement.

3. Budoff, P.W., M.D., *No More Menstrual Cramps and Other Good News*. New York: Penguin, 1981.

   A woman physician writes for women. Budoff is a staunch advocate of women's health and has researched many of the problems herself.

4. Farquhar, J., *The American Way of Life Need Not Be Hazardous to Your Health*. New York: Norton, 1979.

   An invaluable and detailed guide to the behavior modification school of habit change. Gives specific and detailed strategies for progressing in exercise programs, stress management, weight management, and qualitative dietary change.

5. Holvey, D.N., Editor. *The Merck Manual of Diagnosis and Therapy*. Rahway, NJ: Merck Sharp and Dohme Research Laboratories, 1982.

Available in many bookstores. A disease-oriented manual of diagnostic and therapeutic information. Useful if you know, or think you know, what you've got.

6. Kiester, E., Jr., Editor. *Better Homes and Gardens New Family Medical Guide*. Des Moines, Iowa: Better Homes and Gardens Books, 1982.

A very readable, useful and nicely illustrated guide that is focused mostly on disease and illness. A good reference book if you are interested in looking up a particular problem. Also gives normal anatomy and physiology.

7. *Medical Self-Care*, P.O. Box 717, Inverness, CA 94937

A quarterly magazine begun on a shoestring by Tom Ferguson, M.D., and with Sehnert's book, a pioneering effort in self-care. Edited and published by Michael Castelman, Carole Pisarczyk and Ferguson. Has excellent balance of health maintenance and illness care. On most newstands.

8. *Our Bodies, Our Selves*. The Boston Women's Health Book Collective. New York: Simon and Schuster, 1976.

A good and important book. The bible of the women's health movement. For details on the prevention and treatment of illness in women it is the best available.

9. *Prevention Magazine*. Rodale Press, Inc., 33 E. Minor St., Emmaus, PA 18049. (215) 967-5171.

A Rodale publication that gives priority to nutritional and vitamin-based approaches to health. On some newsstands.

10. Roberts, T.M., Tinker, K.M., and Kemper, D.W. *Healthwise Handbook*. New York: Doubleday Dolphin, 1979.

A balanced, nicely illustrated book on the diagnosis, treatment, and prevention of the more common illnesses.

11. Ryan, R.S. and Travis, J.W. *Wellness*

Workbook. Berkeley, CA: Ten Speed Press, 1981.

Along with Ardell and the Healthwise people, Travis was a pioneer of the Wellness movement. This workbook is loaded with exercises for use in attaining the higher levels of wellness.

12. Sehnert, K.W. with Eisenberg, H. *How To Be Your Own Doctor (Sometimes)*. New York: Grossett and Dunlap, 1975.

The first book for "activated" patients and self-care. It deals with both illness care and health maintenance.

13. Sobel, D.S. and Ferguson, T. *The People's Book of Medical Tests*. Summit Books, In Press.

14. Vickery, D. and Fries, J.F. *Take Care of Yourself. A Consumer's Guide to Medical Care*. Reading, MA: Addison-Wesley, 1981.

A very useful book that leads the reader along symptom paths and helps them decide what to do next and when to seek medical care.

15. Werner, D. *Where There Is No Doctor*. The Hesperian Foundation, P.O. Box 1962, Palo Alto, CA., 94302, 1977.

A remarkable "village health-care handbook," written originally in Spanish as a self-care manual for Mexican people with no formal medical care. It is readable, well illustrated, and its focus on disease of a rural, poor subtropical area does not distract from its usefulness as an illness reference in our society.

ORGANIZATIONS

1. Center for Medical Consumers, 237 Thompson Street, New York, N.Y., 10012 (212) 674-7105. This organization is a clearinghouse for medical and health information for consumers. They maintain a library where people can come, get assistance, and read. They will provide special help by mail and over the

phone when requested. In addition, they publish an excellent newsletter, *Health Facts*, 8–12 times a year. It is well researched and written. The center will furnish an index of past issues on request.

2. National Health Information Clearinghouse, P.O. Box 1133, Washington, D.C., 20013. Provides some of the same services as #1.

3. Planetree Health Resource Center, 2040 Webster St., San Francisco, CA., 94115 (415) 346-4636. This center covers medical matters as well as the health and well-being material. It has a library and offers information packets by mail (any drug, any disease, any alternative) for $5.00 and in-depth research packets for $35.00.

4. The Self-Help Center, 1600 Dodge Ave., Suite S-122, Evanston, IL., 60201. ". . . a not-for-profit organization devoted to understanding, forming, and assisting self-help/mutual aid groups nationwide." The center helps existing groups to start new chapters as well as helping form new groups for unmet needs. It also educates health professionals to work with and utilize self-help groups more effectively, and does research on the effectiveness and economic role of self-help groups. It has published a directory of self-help groups in the Chicago area.

Index

Abdomen
  exercises for, 229
  how to examine, 58–59
Aches, alternatives to conventional therapy, 205
Addiction, and habit, 105–106
Additives, and food, 142–143
Adolescence, and the Lifetime Health-Monitoring Plan, 219–220
Adulthood, young, and "Lifetime Health-Monitoring Plan," 220
Advocacy, 95, 96, 98–100
  and health partnerships, 175
  in the hospital, 210–211
Aerobic exercise, 125
AIDS syndrome, 90
Alcohol, 108
  medical consequences of too much, 135
  use questionnaire, 28
Alexander technique, 121
Alignment
  and health, 113–114
  assessing, 114
  assuming good, 114–116
  lifting heavy weights and, 116
  maintaining, 115–116
Anaerobic sports, 125
Anger, 74–76
Antibiotics, and food, 142
Anxiety
  alternatives to conventional therapy, 205–206
  habits and, 106
Appetite
  in relation to different foods, 147–148
  set point, 147
Arms, exercises for, 227–228
Arteriosclerosis
  and diet, 136
  See also Heart attack
Arteriosclerotic heart disease, factors which increase risk of, 26
Assertiveness
  during physician's office visits, 192
  in health partnerships, 177

Backs
  and alignment, 114–116
  lower, exercises for, 228–229
  problems with, 118–120
Balance, muscular, 116–117
Belly
  exercises for, 229
  how to examine, 58–59
Biofeedback, 203–204
Blood pressure, how to measure, 56–57
Body fat, 146–147. See also Fat
Body-mind connection. See Mind-Body Connection
Breslow, Lester, 218–223
Bronchitis. See Respiratory diseases
Buttocks, exercises for, 228–229

Caffeine, 106, 108
Calcium, 135–136
Calf, exercises for, 230
Calories
  and weight management, 149
  consumption of, during exercise (table), 131
  medical consequences of too many, 135
Cancers, 21–24
  and diet, 136
  and imagery, 204
  and mind-body connection, 66–67
  factors which increase risk of, 26
  standard vs. alternative therapy, 176
Challenge, openness to, 20
Chemotherapy, alternatives to, 176
Children, and "Lifetime Health-Monitoring Plan," 219
Choice, and habits, 107
Cholesterol, blood serum, and diet, 136
Chiropractic, 121
Cirrhosis, 21–24
  factors which increase risk of, 26
  See also Liver
Communication
  and health partnerships, 174
  and relationships, 85–86
  in person-doctor relationships, 165–167

Constipation
  alternatives to conventional therapy,
    204–205
  standard vs. alternative therapy, 176
Control, in person-doctor relationships, 162,
    164–165
Coronary artery disease
  and diet, 136
  standard vs. alternative therapy, 176
  See also Heart attack
Counseling, 81–82

"Day-tight" compartments, living in, 76
Death, leading causes of, by population type
    (tables), 21–24
Dependency, 87–88
Diabetes, standard vs. alternative therapy, 176
Diastolic blood pressure readings, 56
Diet
  and disease, 135, 136
  and weight management, 150–151
  typical American, 134–135
  See also Nutrition
Discipline, 80
Diseases, and illnesses, 69–70
Disks, spinal, problems with, 119
Doctor-Patient relationship. *See* Person-Doctor
    relationship
Doctors. *See* Physicians
Drugs, 106, 108
  and addiction, 105–106
  use questionnaire, 28

Ears, how to examine, 57–58
Eating. *See* Nutrition
Eating, moving, and habits, overview,
    103–104
Elderly, and "Lifetime Health-Monitoring
    Plan," 221
Emotional-Spiritual health, 13
  advocacy and people-support, 95–101
  characteristics of, 79–81
  continuum, 78–79
  individual, 72–82
  mind-body connection, 63–71
  overview, 61–62
  questionnaire, 29–30
  relationships, 83–94
Emotions, 74–76
Empathy, 97
Emphysema. *See* Respiratory diseases
Environmental Protection Agency, and food,
    143
Ethylene Dibromide, 143
Exercise(s), 226–231
  aerobic and anaerobic, 125
  and everyday activities, 128–129

and weight management, 148, 150
assessing your activity patterns, 125–128
barriers to, 128
choosing, 131
effects of, 125
getting into it, 131–133
personal profile, 126–127
preparing for, 130
questionnaire, 27
why exercises, 123–125

Fat, 134–138 *passim*
  medical consequences of too much, 135
  See also Body fat; Weight management
Fat is a Feminist Issue (Orbach), 152
Feldenkreis school, 121
Fiber, medical consequences of too little, 135
Fitness, questionnaire, 27
Flexibility, muscular, 116–117
Food, alteration and processing of, 142–143
Food. *See also* Diet; Nutrition

Gibran, Kahlil, *The Prophet*, 74
Globus hystericus, 2
Gratification, delayed, 20, 80
Gregory, Ellen, 120
Grief, and habits, 108–109

Habit and lifestyle questionnaire, 26–31
Habits, 13, 25
  an approach to changing, 109–112
  analyzing, 109–110
  and addictions, 105–106
  and choice, 107
  and health problems or conditions, 106
  changing unhealthy, 105–112
  grieving and, 108–109
  personal benefits of, 108
  unhealthy, 106–107
Health
  definition of, 8, 10–11
  definition of a well person, 76–77
  monitoring, 39–40
  personal goals, 18
  personal planning guide, preparing, 33–36
  personal planning guide, prioritizing, 36–39
  personal, questionnaire, 28
Health accounting, 13
  gathering and describing skills, 52–60
  inventory, 17–32
  overview, 15–16
  personal health guide, 33–40
  self-health record, 41–51
Health care, characteristics of present, 2–4
Health professionals, and the mind-body con-
    nection, 68–69
Heart attack, 21–24

and diet, 136
and mind-body connection, 65–66
factors which increase risk of, 26
habits and, 106
Heart rate, measuring, 130
Herbicides, and food, 142
Heroin, 108
Herpes, genital, 90
High blood pressure. *See* Hypertension
Holistic health, 5, 8, 10
Hospital, being in the, 207–213
Hypertension
    and diet, 135–136
    and mind-body connection, 65–66
    standard vs. alternative therapy, 176

Illness
    and disease, 69–70
    as a teacher, 8, 12
    care of, 13
    emotional, societal dislike of, 2–4
    monitoring and recording, 195
    overview, 155–156
Imagery, 204
Infancy, and "Lifetime Health-Monitoring
    Plan," 219
Insecticides, and food, 142
Insulin, stimulating potential of, by different
    foods, 148
Interdependence, 96
Intimacy, 87–88
Inventory
    emotional-spiritual, 19
    personal health, past and present conditions,
        18–20
    personal health, potential future problems,
        20, 25
Isolation, 95–96, 107

Leg, excercises for, 229–230
Lifestyle, 25
    habit questionnaire, 26–31
"Lifetime Health-Monitoring Plan," 218–223
Listening, 107
    and communication, 85
Liver, habits and, 106
Love, 96
    and communication, 86
    in person-doctor relationships, 169–170

Manipulation, in relationships, 89–90
Massage, 204
Masturbation, 90–91, 92
Medical records
    examining, 51
    obtaining, 44–45, 48–51
    States' status on, 224–225

Medications
    making a list of, 182
    safe use of, 178–183
Medicine, Western, alternatives to, 8, 11
Meditation, 202
Metabolism, altered in fat people, 148
Middle age, and "Lifetime Health-Monitoring
    Plan," 220
Mind-Body connection, 63–71, 10
    and cancers, 66–67
    and health professionals, 68–69
    and heart attack, 65–66
    and hypertension, 65–66
    and the placebo effect, 67–68
    beliefs, 65
Movement
    questionnaire, 27
    See also Exercise
Moving, 13

Neck
    exercises for, 226–227
    problems with, 118, 119–120
Nurses, in the hospital, 211–212
Nutrition, 13
    alternative, 137–139
    comparison of prevalent and alternative,
        (table), 138
    eating habits questionnaire, 26
    medical consequences of unhealth (table),
        135
    principles of good, 136–137
    See also Diet

Office visit, to physician, maximizing the,
    191–197
Orbach, Susie, *Fat is a Feminist Issue*, 152
Osler, William, *A Way of Life*, 76
Osteopathy, 121
Overweight. *See* Weight management

Personal Health Competence, 12–14
    and mind-body relationships, 64–65
    health beliefs of, 8–12
    overview, 1–6
Partnerships, health, 172–183
    skills for, 173–180
    underlying beliefs of, 172–173
Pathways (overviews) of
    eating, moving, and habits, 103–104
    emotional-spiritual health, 61–62
    health accounting and information gather-
        ing, 15–16
    illness and problem care, 155–156
Patients
    rights of, 209
    vs. persons, 157–158

Peck, M. S., *The Road Less Traveled*, 19–20, 80
People-Support systems. *See* Support systems
Perls, Fritz, 121
Person-Doctor relationships, 157–171
  collaborative partnership, 161–162
  communication in, 42, 165–157
  control and responsibility in, 162
  expectations in, 167–168
  love and creativity in, 169–170
  unsatisfactory, 158–160
  See also Partnerships, health; Relationships
Physicians
  and the mind-body connection, 68–69
  choosing, 184–190
  maximizing the office visit to, 191–197
  responsibility of, for your health, 7–8
Placebo effect, 65, 67–68
Posture. *See* Alignment
Pregnancy, and the Lifetime Health-
    Monitoring Plan, 218–219
Prophet, The (Gibran), 74
Pulse
  how to measure, 55–56
  target range for, during exercise, 130–131
Put-Downs, 93–94

Quackery, guarding against, 177–178

Recommended Daily Allowances, 139, 140–141
Records, medical. *See* Medical records
Relationships, 83–94
  and changing others, 89–93
  context of, 86–87
  essentials of, 84–87
  obstacles to, 87–94
  See also Person-Doctor relationships
Relaxation, 202
  questionnaire, 28
Respiration, how to measure, 57
Respiratory diseases
  factors which increase risk of, 26
  standard vs. alternative therapy, 176
Responsibility, for your health, 2, 8, 9–10, 20, 80
  in person-doctor relationships, 162, 164–165
  in physician's office visits, 193–194
Risk factors, for heart attack, 65–66
Road Less Traveled, The (Peck), 19–20, 80
Rolf, Ida, 120
Rolfing, 120
Rubenfeld Synergy, 121
Rubenfeld, Illana, 121

Safety habits, questionnaire, 27
Salt, 135–138 *passim*

medical consequences of too much, 135
Self-Awareness, 52–53
Self-Esteem, 79
Self-Health record
  benefits of, 42–43
  flowsheet, 48
  in the hospital, 210
  preparing, 43–45
  progress record in, 46–49
Sex, and sexuality, 90–93
Shoulders
  exercises for, 227–228
  problems with, 119–120
Sickness. *See* Illness
Skin, how to examine, 58
Smoking, 106, 107, 108
  questionnaire, 29
Soma Neuromuscular Integration, 120
Somers, Ann, 218–223
Spine, and alignment, 114–116
Spirituality, active, 72–74
Sports. *See* Anaerobic sports *and* Exercise(s)
Stress
  alternatives to conventional therapy, 205–206
  and heart attack, 66
  injuries from, 116–117
  questionnaire, 28
Strokes, 21–24
  factors which increase rise of, 26
Sugar, 135–138 *passim*
  insulin stimulating potentional of, 148
  medical consequences of too much, 135
Support, and communication, 86
Support groups, 98
Support networks, 98
Support systems
  and habits, 109
  characteristics of People-, 97–99
  for weight management, 150
  problems, 100–101
  See also Advocacy
Surgery, alternatives to, 8, 11, 175–176
Systolic blood pressure readings, 56

Temperature, how to take, 54–55
Tension
  alternatives to conventional therapy, 205–206
  target zone, 63
Therapy, 81–82
  alternative to conventional, 198–206
  groups, 98
  standard vs. alternative, 176
Thigh, excercises for, 230–231
Throat, how to examine, 57
Tooth care, 106

Touching, 97

Vascular lesions of central nervous system. *See* Strokes
Vitamins, 139–141

Walking
  and alignment, 15
  as exercise, 129
Way of Life, A (Osler), 76
Weight management
  and body fat, 144–153
  and diet, 150–151

and exercise, 148, 150
and women, 151–152
facts about, 148–150
guidelines for losing weight, 150–151
ideal weight tables, 146
what is overweight?, 146–147
Wellness, definition of, 76–77
Wholistic health. *See* Holistic health
Williams, Bill, 120
Women, and weight management, 151–152
Worry, alternatives to conventional therapy, 205–206

Yoga, 115, 117, 120, 202–203